The Common Nature of Epidemics and Their Relation to Climate and Civilization

Thomas Southwood-Smith

Writat

This edition published in 2021

ISBN : 9789390439942

Design and Setting By
Writat
(An Imprint of Vij Publishiing Group)
www.vijbooks.in
contact@vijpublishing.com

Contents

INTRODUCTION

The recent very serious outbreak of Epidemic disease among the cattle in England may not unreasonably induce the fear that a human Epidemic is approaching. Cholera has prevailed in Paris and several other places on the Continent during the late autumn, and it is well known that the former visitations of that terrible disease in this country have appeared the year following similar attacks abroad. Moreover, human epidemics in numerous instances have been preceded or accompanied by extensive murrain among cattle.[1]

1. See pp. 7, 65, 110.

Never was a country guided through the perils of an Epidemic with greater wisdom and energy than Great Britain during the Cholera of 1848–9. The master spirit on that occasion was Dr Southwood Smith. Long previous to that time this great man had had a more extended experience of the nature, causes, and treatment of Zymotic diseases than perhaps any physician before or since. He had made them his special study, and applied the great powers of his clear, reasoning, and philosophic mind, to the discovery of their causes, and the best means of arresting their progress.

Whilst occupying the post of responsibility as the chief medical adviser of the nation in his capacity of Medical Member of the General Board of Health, Dr Southwood Smith left behind him a set of official reports on the subjects of Epidemics, Contagion, and Quarantine, which will never die.

"The reports drawn up by Dr Southwood Smith," writes Dean Peacock, "on the proper precautions to be taken to meet the recent outbreaks of cholera, have been of the most essential service wherever their recommendations have been followed. If Dr S. Smith, however, had no other claims on the lasting gratitude of the nation, I would refer to his reports on quarantine, as quite sufficient to establish them. They have contributed, more than any other publications on this subject, to dissipate the gross and mischievous delusions upon which these regulations are founded, and which are known to be so injurious to the free commercial intercourse and prosperity of nations."

After Dr Southwood Smith left office he gave us a concise summary of his experience in two masterly lectures, now published, together with extracts from his official Reports.

In times of distress it is only natural to look for the most efficient help. Our herds only have extensively suffered of late, but we ourselves may follow, and it is well to be prepared. Even with reference to the causes and treatment of the Epizootic, the reasonings, facts, and conclusions again brought forward in the following pages will apply. But should the worst fears become realized, and an extensive human epidemic follow, these writings will tell with greater force, and the nation will be better prepared to meet the danger, for having calmly considered beforehand the probability of its approach.

***

One ground of hope that we may escape a visitation of Cholera during the coming summer, may be afforded by the remarkably tempestuous weather which prevailed in December and January last.[2] The loss of the steam-ship "London," which foundered in the Bay of Biscay, with 226 souls, on the 11th January, and the still more remarkable fact, that during the night of the 10th, out of 62 vessels riding at anchor in Torbay, 41 either foundered or were dashed to pieces on the rocks;—these were terrible calamities, and they were only the most striking examples of the numerous wrecks and disasters which occurred in the course of the late most tempestuous season;—but they afford a hope of escape from a worse peril, viz. nations prostrated by disease and premature death.

T. B.

KINGSCOTE, WOKINGHAM,

May, 1866.

2. See p. 18.

THE COMMON NATURE

OF

EPIDEMICS

Some account of the structure and functions of the human frame, of the action of physical agents on this wonderful machinery, and of the principles which relate to Individual, as well as to Public Health, ought to form a part of elemental education. There is a growing conviction that the necessity for such knowledge is not restricted to the physician; that it is essential also to the educator, the mother, the nurse, and indeed to every one who would enjoy, together with the due development of his physical, intellectual, and moral nature, the full term of the boon of life.

The main causes which shorten and embitter human life, as far as that unhappy result depends on the disturbance of health, are within our own control. There is the closest connection between the knowledge we have acquired of the physical conditions on which the life and health of individuals and communities depend, and on our command over those conditions. Every fact we have learnt respecting the great laws of nature, on our conformity to which our very existence depends, has taught us that the circumstances which produce excessive sickness and early death are preventible.

The character of Pestilence which gave it its great power and terror—that it walketh in darkness,—is its character no longer. Its veil has fallen, and with it its strength. A clear and steady light now marks its course from its commencement to its end; and that light places in equally broad and strong relief its antagonist and conqueror—CLEANLINESS.

*****

The term Epidemic has become a popular one. It is derived from two Greek words, which signify "upon the people—prevalent among the people"—diseases which, at one and the same time, prevail extensively among large masses of the people.

Recently these diseases have received another name, which is also becoming familiar—"Zymotic," from a Greek word, which signifies to "ferment," as if the efficient cause of these diseases, whatever it may be, acts in the manner of a ferment.

Epidemic diseases, though called by a common name, present great differences in their external characters. Plague, Yellow Fever, Cholera, Small-Pox, Typhus, Scarlet Fever, Influenza, present characters so definite and special, that they have been naturally regarded as distinct diseases, and they really are so different as to render it desirable, for many reasons, that each should be discriminated and denoted by its proper name. Amidst this great diversity in form, however, they present very striking resemblances, of which the following are generally recognized:—

1. Epidemics resemble each other in being all fevers. They all exhibit that particular assemblage of symptoms which from time immemorial it has been agreed to denote by the term Fever.

This is as true of the great Epidemics of former times as of those which prevail in our own.

The so-called Black Death of the 14th century was a fever—an aggravated form of the Oriental or Bubo-Plague; in which there occurred, in addition to the ordinary symptoms of that dreadful disease, effusions of black blood, forming black spots on the arms, face, and chest. From this circumstance it derived its name. These effusions on the external surface of the body were accompanied by profuse and mortal discharges from the internal organs.

The Oriental Plague, the great devastator of Europe in former times, and still the scourge of some portions of it, is a fever characterized by specific glandular inflammation.

The Sweating Sickness of the 15th and 16th centuries was a fever, with symptoms of acute rheumatism, attended with a fœtid perspiration which poured from the body in streams. "Suddenly," says Hollingshed, "a deadly burning sweat assailed their bodies and distempered their blood, and all, as soon as the sweat took them, yielded the ghost."

The Cholera of modern times is a fever, which appears in its true character when the first stroke of the disease does not prove fatal, and time is allowed for the full development of its successive stages.

The common Epidemics of the day—Ordinary as distinguished from Extraordinary Epidemics—typhus, scarlet fever, small-pox, measles,—are so universally recognized as fevers that the popular notion of fever is derived from the external characters which these maladies present.

2. Epidemics resemble each other in the extent of their range. Ordinary diseases attack single individuals, and if, from season or other causes, several cases occur simultaneously, they are still isolated and scattered. They

never prevail at the same time among several members of a family, or among the inhabitants generally of a court, street, or town. Epidemics, on the contrary, derive their name from their attacking large numbers at once.

The great Epidemics of all ages have been strikingly characterized by their wide-spread course. The Black Death extended from China to Greenland, and desolated in its course Asia, Europe, and Africa.

The Bubo-Plague of the middle ages often extended beyond its proper seat. In the 15th century it spread seventeen times over different European countries, and extended to the most distant northern nations.

The Sweating Sickness prevailed simultaneously or in rapid succession over England, France, Germany, Prussia, Poland, Russia, Norway, and Sweden. "It extended," say the chronicles of the day, "like a violent conflagration which spread in all directions; yet the flames did not issue from one focus, but rose up everywhere as if self-ignited."

The Influenza of the middle ages took a range which may be said to have been universal. In our own day we have seen the same disease attack almost every family, in nearly every city, town, and village; spread within a short period over the whole of Europe, and then extend through the vast continent of the New World.

Cholera traverses the earth in zones, spreads with equal facility through tropical and polar regions, and attacks alike the seats of civilization and the huts of the slave and the savage.

3. Epidemics resemble each other in the rapidity of their course. Sometimes, indeed, they begin slowly, advance haltingly, and gather strength in silence. For some time they give so little indication of their power that the apprehension of their presence is very constantly regarded as a "false alarm." Now and then, here and there, they strike a sudden and mortal blow; but it is only an individual that falls. After a considerable interval, perhaps at a great distance, another blow is struck; and then one by one, another and another, until at last the fact becomes too manifest to be doubted or denied, that two victims have been seized in one family— several in the same street—three or four on the same day, in distant parts of the town, or in the adjoining town, or it may be in towns separated from each other by the distance of hundreds of miles. At length the terror-stricken nation, startled from its fondly cherished security, sees no place safe from the Plague. When, however, the causes are intense, it may break forth quite suddenly, and spread with astonishing rapidity.

In 1831, when Cholera first appeared in Cairo, it extended within the space of five days over the whole of Lower Egypt, desolating simultaneously all the towns and villages of the Delta.

In 1832 it leaped at one bound from London to Paris, and when once there, spread in five days over thirty-five out of forty-eight quarters of the city.

When Influenza broke out in London in 1847, it spread in one day over every part of the metropolis, and upwards of 500,000 persons suffered from the malady.

4. Epidemics resemble each other in giving distinct and unmistakeable warnings of their approach. These warnings consist of two events: first, the sudden outbreak and general spread of some milder epidemic; and, secondly, the transformation of ordinary diseases into diseases of a new type, more or less resembling the character of the extraordinary disease at hand.

It is a very singular fact that both in the middle ages, and in modern times, the lesser Epidemic which has generally preceded and pre-announced the coming of the greater, is Influenza.

The history of European Epidemics from the 14th century downwards, shows that whenever a new Plague was at hand, destined to become truly European, it was preceded by a sudden outbreak of Influenza, as general as it was violent. This is exemplified with singular uniformity in the Epidemics of the 16th century—the severest epidemic period on record. It is most remarkable that in our own day the first visitation of Epidemic Cholera was preceded by an outbreak of Influenza which resembled, in the most minute particulars, the violent and universal Influenza that ushered in the mortal Sweating Sickness Epidemic of 1517.

So again, on the second visitation of Cholera, in 1848, it was preceded, as we have just seen, by the universal Influenza of 1847.[3]

> <u>3</u>. It may be remarked that for some time prior to the Cattle Plague in the autumn of 1865, the disease called *pleuro-pneumonia* had extensively prevailed among the herds throughout the country. [ED.]

The second circumstance, and a most instructive one it is, premonitory of the advent of a great Epidemic, is a general transformation of the type of ordinary diseases into the characteristic type of the approaching pestilence. Sydenham gives a graphic description of such a transformation in the character of the fevers and inflammatory diseases prevailing in London some months before the outbreak of the Great Plague. He states that this change consisted in an approximation, in several striking features, of the general type of disease, to the distinguishing characters of the Pestilence which had not yet appeared, but was close at hand.

In 1831, in the wards of the London Fever Hospital, I observed and recorded a precisely similar change in the general type of the fevers in London, six months before the first visitation of Cholera. Anterior to that period, fever in London, for a long series of years, had been essentially an acute, inflammatory disease, for which bloodletting and other depleting remedies were indispensable. At this period it ceased to be an inflammatory disease; it became a disease of debility, in which no one could think of bleeding; and so closely did the prevailing fever now put on the general character of the approaching plague, which was as yet six months distant, that the fever into which those Cholera patients fell, who were not killed by the first stroke—the consecutive fever, as it was afterwards called—could not be distinguished from the primary fever in the wards of the Hospital when Cholera was at its height, which had appeared there for the first time six months previously, and which has never disappeared since.[4]

4. This was written in November, 1855.

It is further very remarkable that the Professors of Veterinary Medicine and Surgery in London noted at the same time a similar change in the type of the diseases of the lower animals—horses, cows, sheep, and all domestic creatures;—a change requiring a similar modification of the remedies which they had been in the habit of using.

5. A further character of great Epidemics, partly arising from the last, is this:—they are actually present and in operation some time before they assume their distinct and proper form. Sometimes, indeed, the very first cases are most intense and characteristic, but at others they are scarcely to be distinguished from the severer attacks of ordinary disease of a like nature. Hence doubt is sometimes reasonably entertained of their true character. When at length increasing numbers leave no doubt of the actual presence of the dreaded malady, the first announcement of it is always received with incredulity and sometimes with resentment; and so it is that Epidemics always take a country by surprise—burst suddenly on an unprepared people, who wilfully shut their eyes against the plainest evidence, as if they would avert the event by denying its existence.

6. Again, Epidemics resemble each other in the uniformity of their course. They present, with great regularity, periods of comparative quiescence and activity—periods of well-marked increase, culmination, and decrease.

7. They further resemble each other in the manner of their migration. They advance by leaps. On breaking out in a locality they soon come to their height, decline, and disappear. Then they attack another locality; here they pass through precisely the same process as before, and proceed to a third, fourth, or fifth district, and so on. Sometimes indeed they localize themselves on the same spot for a considerable period, and then several places may be simultaneously affected; but for the most part a large city may be regarded as a cluster of towns, through the several districts of which epidemics advance as if they were proceeding from one town or village to another. Hence the duration of an epidemic in a place is generally proportionate to its size. The several localities attacked being visited in succession, a space of time is required to spread through the whole of them proportionate to the magnitude of the town.

8. Epidemics resemble each other in the periodicity of their return.

On its first visitation (1485) the Sweating Sickness spread over the whole of England in the course of one year, when it disappeared.

After an interval of twenty years it broke out a second time quite suddenly (1505); revisited nearly all the seats of its former ravages, and again disappeared at the end of six months.

On its third visitation (1517), after an interval of eleven years, it again finished its course within six months.

Its fourth visitation (1528) was repeated after a further interval of precisely eleven years. Such was its violence on this occasion, that the historians of that day designate this period by the significant name of the "Great Mortality." It drove Henry VIII. from London, destroyed several of the most distinguished persons of the Court, impressed the nation, from the monarch to the peasant, with an awful feeling of the uncertainty of life, continued its destructive course for its accustomed period of six months, and then again disappeared.

From this to its fifth and last visitation, twenty-three years elapsed (from 1528 to 1551.) It then broke out with unmitigated fury, spread once more over the whole of England, ceased within six months, and from that period has never reappeared in any country.

The Oriental Plague of the middle ages returned with a like periodicity; and so it does at the present day in the countries in which it maintains its ancient reign. It recurs with much regularity about every ten years.

The Fever Epidemics of the metropolis return pretty constantly about every ten or twelve years.

The Irish Typhus Epidemics have recurred nearly decennially for the last 150 years.

Epidemic Cholera, on its first visitation, ravaged Great Britain for a period of fifteen months. It then wholly ceased; after an interval of sixteen years it again broke out, and pursued its former course for the same exact period of fifteen months, and then ceased.

Within the brief interval of only five years, it last year (1854) accomplished its third visitation. It now protracted its stay for a period of seventeen months; coming sooner and staying longer.

9. Again, Epidemics resemble each other in the brevity of the space that intervenes between the attack and death.

The Black Death was often fatal on the first day of the attack—generally on the third or fourth. In England it was sometimes fatal within twelve hours, and frequently in two days, particularly when spitting of blood or any other form of hœmorrhage was amongst the early symptoms.

The violent inflammatory fever which characterized the Sweating Sickness, generally ran its course in a few hours; in severe cases, indeed, the crisis was always over within a day and night, but it often proved fatal in six hours.

In our own day we have witnessed many instances in which Epidemic Cholera was fatal within twelve hours. I have known several in which the fatal event followed in ten hours, the patient having been within an hour of the dreaded attack in *apparent* health.

In all great epidemics the protraction of the disease beyond three or four days is a favourable omen. One of the objects in the treatment of the sick is to gain time. If Nature's first violent effort to expel the enemy that has taken possession of the system, does not destroy life, the vital powers rally, and the frame often survives the storm.

10. Lastly, Epidemics resemble each other in being produced by the same causes. The whole tenor of experience shows that whatever produces an especial liability to one epidemic, produces a similar liability to every other.

The Causes of epidemics, as of all other diseases, are divided into two classes,—the predisposing and the primary. The predisposing causes are those circumstances which bring the body into a fit state for the action of the primary. The primary cause is the agent which directly and immediately excites the disease.

If a number of persons, in an ordinary state of health, say a hundred, are exposed to the primary cause of any epidemic—to the poison of Cholera for example—probably not more than ten would be seized with the disease. Why do the ninety escape? The poison, by the supposition, encompasses and acts upon all alike: why do ten only suffer? Suppose these same hundred persons took a large dose of arsenic, or an over-dose of chloroform, not only would not one in ten escape, but every individual would certainly perish.

It is conceived that the primary cause cannot take effect unless the system be in a state of susceptibility to its action; that there is in the body an innate power of resistance to all noxious agents of this kind, rendering it, when in full vigour, invulnerable to them; that there are certain circumstances which weaken or destroy this resisting power, and which even impart to the body a peculiar susceptibility to the influence of such agents—and these circumstances are called predisposing causes.

The predisposing causes of epidemics may be divided into two classes— External and Internal. The external are those which vitiate the atmosphere; the internal are those which more immediately vitiate the blood.

The vitiators of the atmosphere include overcrowding, filth, putrescent animal and vegetable matters of all kinds, exhalations from foul cesspools, sewers, rivers, canals, ditches, marshes, swamps, &c. Causes of this class are also called *localizing,* because they favour the generation and spread of epidemics in the localities in which they abound.

The causes which more immediately act from within are those which either directly introduce pernicious matters into the interior of the body, in the shape of foul water or putrescent food; or which indirectly accumulate noxious matters within the system, by impairing the action of the excretory or depurating organs whose office it is to maintain the blood in a state of purity, by removing out of the system substances which having served their purpose have become useless and pernicious.

The earnest attention which has been recently directed to the first class of causes has led to an advancement in the science of prevention, the importance of which it is impossible to over-estimate.

To give only one illustration of the action of a predisposing cause, I select as my example, *Overcrowding.*

The Statistical Society of London some time ago appointed a Committee of its Council to make a house-to-house examination of the parish of Marylebone, with a view to ascertain how many families in the parish occupied a single room as a living and sleeping room. In the course of this inquiry, one of the examiners came to a house in which there was one remarkable room. It was occupied not by one family only, but by five. A separate family ate, drank, and slept in each of the four corners of this room; a fifth occupied the centre.

"But how can you exist," said the visitor to a poor woman whom he found in the room (the other inmates being absent on their several avocations), "how can you possibly exist?"

"Oh, indeed, your honour," she replied, "we did very well until the gentleman in the middle took in a lodger."

I see every day in the wards of the Fever Hospital the consequence of taking in such lodgers. An epidemic shows it not more truly, but more strikingly.

Within the walls of an establishment for pauper children at Tooting, in 1849, there were crowded 1395 children. Little more than one hundred cubic feet of breathing space was allowed for each child, 500 being the smallest compatible with safety. One night Cholera attacked sixty-four of these children; 300 were attacked in all. Within a week 180 perished.

In the Workhouse of Taunton there were 276 inmates. In some of the rooms the breathing space was not more than sixty-eight cubic feet. Cholera swept away 60 of these inhabitants in less than a week.

In the County Jail of this same town, the breathing space allowed to each prisoner ranges from 819 to 935 cubic feet. Not a single case of cholera, nor even of diarrhœa, occurred among the prisoners in this jail.

The town's people also escaped, while in the overcrowded workhouses, 22 per cent. of the total number of the inhabitants were swept away.

In the village of East Farleigh, near Maidstone, 1000 persons were assembled for hop-picking. They were lodged in sheds, and had about eighty cubic feet for breathing space: in a few days diarrhœa became universal among them: ninety-seven were attacked with cholera, and forty-six died. In the same village, at the same time, under another employer who had provided proper accommodation for his labourers, there was a complete immunity from the epidemic.

I could add cases of the like kind without number. I could show that animals are affected by this cause of disease no less than men; that horses overcrowded in stables die of glanders; dogs in overcrowded kennels die of distemper; sheep overcrowded in ships, even during a short passage from one country to another, die in great numbers of febrile diseases:[5] results which prove the operation of a general law of nature. I could adduce equally decisive examples of the action of each of the principal external predisposing causes just enumerated.

It has been often said that we cannot tell the difference between the air of the mountain-side and that of the crowded hospitals and fever-nests of towns. If it were so, it would be sufficient to say, Life is a more delicate test than Chemistry. But it is not so. The impurities in these pernicious places can be detected by chemical analysis, and examined as readily as the constituents of the atmosphere itself.

> 5. It has been alleged that the Cattle Plague owed its existence to these among perhaps other kindred causes, and human Epidemics have frequently been preceded or accompanied by a murrain among Cattle. See p. 7, and Boa Vista fever, *pot.* [ED.]

The moisture in the air of a crowded room may be condensed by ice. It condenses indeed spontaneously on the walls and windows, and on all surfaces, and may be collected in sufficient quantity for examination and experiment.

If a portion of this deposit be put on a piece of platinum and burnt, a strong odour of organic substance is given off, and a quantity of charcoal remains. If the deposit be allowed to stand for a few days, it forms a solid, thick, glutinous mass, having a strong odour of animal matter. If examined by a microscope, it is seen to undergo a remarkable change. First of all, it is converted into a vegetable growth, and this is followed by the production of multitudes of animalcules,—a decisive proof that it must contain organic matter, otherwise it could not nourish organic beings.[6]

> 6. See the interesting experiments of Dr Angus Smith, on the Air and Water of Towns, "Report of the British Association for the Advancement of Science," p. 16, *et seq.*

At every expiration the lungs pour a portion of organic matter into the surrounding atmosphere; at every moment the skin does the same. This matter is the dead portion of the body, which it is one of the special offices of these depurating organs to remove out of the living system as useless and pernicious.

It is indeed pernicious, for it is an animal poison, more concentrated in this than in any other form of excrementitious matter, since in other excretions the noxious particles, in their transmission out of the body, are diluted with other substances, but as they issue from the lungs and skin, they are in a great degree undiluted. Ventilation and cleanliness prevent this matter from accumulating, and render it innoxious. But it collects in large quantities on the furniture and walls of dirty houses, and is the main cause of the disagreeable smell of the rooms in which it abounds. In some instances the walls are coated with it. It was so in one particular building in which, during a local epidemic outbreak, twelve persons were attacked with cholera, and four died.

From recent chemical and microscopical examinations of the air of some crowded and filthy localities in the metropolis, it appears as a general result, that decomposing organic matter is always contained in such air,—the never-failing presence of animalcules testifying its existence, and their number and size indicating its amount.

Imagine the state of the atmosphere in the dormitories of the Tooting children: in the sixty-eight cubic feet of breathing space of the inmates of the Taunton Workhouse; in the eighty cubic feet of the Kentish hop-pickers; in the four corners and centre of the five-family room.

Conceive the state of the atmosphere in this room at night; all the members of the several families, collected; every breath of external air excluded; the windows, and perhaps even the chimney, carefully fastened up. This stagnant and poisoned air, breathed over and over again by every individual for seven or eight hours continuously; respiration, the special and admirable apparatus which nature has constructed for purifying the blood, thus made the very means of corrupting it. I have known from two to three cases of typhus produced nightly, for a fortnight together, in a room of this description, by sleeping in it for a single night! Can we wonder at the generation of typhus in such a room in *ordinary* seasons! Can we wonder at the spread and the havoc of an epidemic in it in *epidemic* seasons?

***

But besides the contamination of the air by external causes, it is conceived that the atmosphere itself undergoes natural changes which predispose it to the development and spread of epidemics. From time immemorial, the popular belief has been that such changes do take place, and that they manifest themselves by unmistakeable signs.

Among such signs may be reckoned,—a disturbance of the regular and ordinary condition of the atmosphere; an inversion of the seasons— summer in winter, and winter in summer; long-continued drought succeeded by torrents of rain, causing rivers to overflow, and the seed to rot in the earth; cloud, mist, fog, favouring excessive dampness, under the influence of which spring up inordinate growths of the lower species of plants, producing mouldiness, and the blood-spots, and other coloured vegetation that adhere to houses, and household furniture, and wearing apparel, and personal ornaments, and the person itself; under which also, fostered by a steadily elevated temperature, spring into being and activity, myriads of the lower tribes of animals—locusts, caterpillars, flies,[7] frogs, covering the face of the earth, and devouring every green thing that the deluge of rain had left; and, as the sequence of these antecedent conditions, dearth and famine, closing the long series of the year's calamities. Such, in all ages and countries, have been the recognized portents and precursors of a coming year of pestilence.

   7. During the autumn following the extraordinary summer of 1865, and in which the Cattle Plague appeared, there was a very marked preponderance of insect life as compared with ordinary seasons. It is asserted by Mr Mc Dougall, of Manchester, that no case of this plague is known to have occurred where his disinfectant, which arrests decomposition, had been freely applied to and about the cattle. [ED.]

And there is truth in this.

It is quite certain that such atmospheric changes do take place, and prepare the way for pestilence. It is quite certain that there is an epidemic meteorology. This epidemic condition of the atmosphere is at length coming within the range of science. The first step towards this result, which promises to be of the highest practical value, we owe to the well-devised and patient observations of Mr Glashier, continued through the three recent Cholera epidemics.

Among other important facts, he has determined that there is—1. An increased pressure of the atmosphere, greatest at the worst period of the epidemic.

2. An increased density of the atmosphere, not arising from an increase of watery vapour; for,

3. The quantity of water in the air was 1/20th less than the average, at the same time that the mean weight of a cubic foot of air was 2 grains above the average.

4. An unusual alternation of heat and cold, yet the heat predominating to such an extent that in particular localities it rose as much as from 2° to 8° above the average. These excesses were most striking at night, particularly in the parts of London on a level with the Thames, where the night temperatures ranged from 7°, 8°, 9°, and 10° above the temperature of the

country, and even of the suburban districts. These temperatures were highest, especially the night ones, when the mortality was greatest; and the mortality was greatest where the temperatures were highest.

5. A remarkable increase above the average in the temperature of the water of the Thames. From a long series of observations it had been found that the normal temperature of the Thames is 51.7°. During the prevalence of the epidemic it rose to 60°, 66°, and once to 70°. At this temperature the "simmering" water must have poured enormous quantities of vapour into the surrounding atmosphere; not the pure vapour of water, for that cannot arise from a river which is the recipient of the foul contents of all the sewers and cesspools of the metropolis. In some instances there was an excess of 20° of the temperature of the water above that of the air. For twenty-eight continuous nights during the height of the epidemic, the average excess exceeded 16.5°.

6. An unusual prevalence of haze, mist, and fog; the fog being sometimes so dense that London could not be discerned from Greenwich.

7. An extraordinary stillness and stagnation of the air, both by day and night. Sometimes in the low-lying districts not a breath could be observed. Even when at more elevated stations the wind was moving with a force of 1 lb 7 oz., the pressure was only ¼ lb in the heart of London.

Wind is the ventilator of nature. Artificial ventilation, as far as it is successful, is an imitation of nature's process. It is stated on undoubted authority (Maitland's History of London) that for several weeks before the Great Plague broke out in London, there was an uninterrupted calm, so that there was not sufficient motion of the air to stir a vane. Baynard, a contemporary physician, confirms this fact. The like circumstance is mentioned by Diemerbroeck in giving an account of the plague at Nimeguen. At the period when the last plague visited Vienna, according to Sir Gilbert Blane, there had been no wind for three months. The terrific outbreak of the cholera at Kurrachee was preceded for some days by such a stagnation of the atmosphere that an oppression scarcely to be endured affected the whole population. It is obvious that calms must favour the accumulation and concentration of effluvia from every source from which they arise.

8. A general deficiency in the tension of common positive electricity.

9. A deficiency of one fourth of the rain-fall for the year. During 118 consecutive days there was scarcely any rain, and not a single drop for 18 days at the period of the highest mortality.

10. A total absence of ozone at all the stations near the river, while at stations of high elevation it was of general occurrence.

These observations relate particularly to the epidemic of 1854, which was more carefully watched than the two former; but the results are similar for each.

"The three epidemics," says Mr Glashier, in summing up the results of his inquiry, "were attended with a particular state of atmosphere, characterized by a prevalent mist, thin in high places, dense in low. During the height of the epidemic, in all cases, the reading of the barometer was remarkably high, the atmosphere thick; and in 1849 and 1854 the temperature above its average. A total absence of rain, and a stillness of air amounting almost to calm, accompanied the progress of the disease on each occasion. In places near the river, the night temperatures were high, with small diurnal range, with a dense torpid mist and air charged with the many impurities arising from the exhalations of the Thames, and adjoining marshes; a deficiency of electricity, and, as shown in 1854, a total absence of ozone, most probably destroyed by the decomposition of the organic matter with which the air in these situations is so strongly charged.

"In both 1849 and 1854, the first decline of the disease was marked by a decrease in the readings of the barometer, and in the temperature of the air and water; the air, which previously had for a long time continued calm, was succeeded by a strong S. W. wind, which soon dissipated the former stagnant and poisonous atmosphere."

We knew before that such influences were in operation, but they had not been weighed and measured. We now know definitely something of an epidemic atmosphere, and the information obtained is most significant; for it shows that the several meteorological changes that take place during the prevalence of an epidemic concur to produce a heavy, warm, moist, and stagnant atmosphere, with disturbed electricity: conditions highly favourable to the decomposition of organic matter.

Under the influence of such an atmosphere, over the moist and warmed surface of every filthy place, over the entire mass of all accumulations of filth in streets, lanes, and courts, and within and about houses, and over the heated surface of all foul water, decomposition goes on with the utmost activity, and the products are poured into the stagnant air.

Against such products the human body has no defence. The lungs admit whatever is brought to them—poisonous and salubrious substances alike. They are guarded by none of those protective contrivances which we see in some other parts of the body. Whatever is capable of suspension in the respired air passes with it directly into the current of the circulation, and when once there, is carried with astonishing rapidity into the very substance of the vital organs.

From the quantity of air which the lungs receive, some conception may be formed of the amount of obnoxious matter which may be introduced into the system through these portals.

At each inspiration there enter the lungs of an ordinary-sized person about 20 cubic inches of air. There are 20 respirations in a minute: 400 cubic inches of air must therefore enter in one minute; 14 cubic feet in one hour, and 366 cubic feet, or 36 hogsheads, in one day. To meet this the heart sends into the lungs at each contraction two ounces of blood; there are 75 pulsations in a minute, during which 150 ounces are propelled into the lungs; a quantity which gives 562 pounds in one hour and 24 hogsheads in 24 hours.

The main purpose for bringing these enormous quantities of air and blood together, with such velocity, is to provide for the enormous waste which is caused by the rapid and unceasing mutation of organic matter. The activity of an organ is sustained at the expense of the matter of which it is composed. No thought passes through the mind, but an equivalent portion of the substance of the brain is consumed; no nervous current flows along the nervous conducters, but a corresponding portion of nervous tissue is used up; no muscular movement, no glandular secretion, takes place without a proportionate waste of muscle and of gland. What must be the amount of supply required to meet this waste, when able-bodied men employed in their ordinary labour lose from 2 lbs. to 5 lbs. and upwards of their weight twice a day.[8] Some physiologists of eminence have estimated that in order to supply that waste, there passes in the course of every 24 hours as much fluid through the thoracic duct[9] as equals the whole quantity of blood in the body.

8. See Experiments on the daily loss of weight sustained by workmen employed in gas-works.—*Philosophy of Health*, 11th Edit. p. 284, *et seq.*

9. The tube which conveys the debris of the body, together with the nutritious part of the food,—both measures of change or waste.

The results of the highly interesting experiments recently made by Professor Graham on the part taken by the active agent in all these processes—organic membrane, of which the organic cell is the type, demonstrates that all the phenomena known as Endosmose and Exosmose depend on a chemical action involving the destruction of organic membrane. In this process chemical action is set up dependent upon active chemical agents, neutral substances being inoperative. Out of this chemical action a new force is induced, the *Osmotic* force; a purely chemical being converted into an equivalent mechanical force, which is made subservient to the essential phenomena of organic and animal life: a *vis motrix*, a force which is to the extra-vascular movements of the body, what the contraction of the heart is to the vascular.

In a frame so constructed, any particles contaminating the circulating fluid most rapidly pervade and contaminate every part of the system.

It has been sometimes imagined that the quantity of matter suspended in the atmosphere and conveyed into the system in respired air, must be too minute to exert any serious influence upon the body.

One single puncture of the finger, so small as not to be visible without the aid of a lens, has introduced into the system a sufficient quantity of putrid matter to cause death with the most violent symptoms.

A few drops of the liquid matter obtained by a condensation of the air of a foul locality, introduced into the vein of a dog, is stated to have produced death with the usual phenomena of typhus fever.

It is certain that on the introduction into the body of an inappreciable portion of the matter of cow-pox, or of small-pox, those specific forms of fever are produced.

From these and similar facts it is inferred, that when putrescent or decomposing organic matter is introduced into the blood it acts as a poison and produces the phenomena of fever, and that all the predisposing causes of epidemics act in this way—by overcharging the blood with the products of decomposing organic matter.

Strictly speaking, however, all that we really know is this—that where certain conditions exist, epidemics break out and spread; that where those conditions do not exist, epidemics do not break out and spread; and that where those conditions did exist, but have been removed, thereupon epidemics cease.

We call those conditions Causes, Predisposing or Localizing Causes, but how they act, whether by accumulating decomposing organic matter in the blood, or in what other way, we have no certain knowledge.

One further fact however is ascertained, that where any one of these predisposing causes is present, epidemics break out and spread just as readily as when all are present together.

Where there is overcrowding alone, for example, epidemics break out and spread. Where there is decomposing filth alone, epidemics break out and spread; and so of the whole number. The removal of one of these causes, therefore, or the removal of two or three of them, will not suffice for safety; every one must be removed before there can be safety.

This we know; all beyond this is conjecture, but as to the most probable of these conjectures, some who have thought on this subject believe that the preponderance of evidence justifies the conclusion that the predisposing causes may themselves become efficient causes; that instances in which they actually do so, are constantly passing before our eyes; that it is practicable to manufacture fever and even epidemic fever to any amount by placing a population under certain known conditions; that it is practicable to prevent the outbreak of epidemics altogether by placing the population under certain other conditions;[10] that the prevalence of the predisposing causes in particular localities, in certain intensities, is sufficient to produce local epidemic outbreaks; that the prevalence of such causes in such intensities, joined to some general conditions of the atmosphere, such as the meteorological conditions which have been enumerated, particularly those which favour the accumulation and concentration of the products of organic decomposition, are all that is required to engender wide-spread epidemics. Those who adopt this view contend that the existence of a primary cause as a distinct and separate entity is not necessary to account for the phenomena.

The more common opinion however is, that joined to the predisposing causes there must always be present a primary cause, having a distinct existence, capable of travelling from one part of the globe to another; capable of spreading over any space however extended, or of confining itself to any space however small—a district, a street, a house, a room.

10. See Baltimore case, p. 78.

It is urged that though we are unacquainted with the physical form or chemical properties of this body, this is no reason why we should not understand its force as a special agent in the production of disease, just as we know the forces of other physical bodies, though not their nature.

The existence of such a body being assumed, it is conceived that it exists not in a gaseous but in a liquid state. It is supposed that it cannot exist in a gaseous state because a gas is readily diffused and dissipated; because when organic matter is reduced to a gaseous state, it has passed from the organic into the inorganic kingdom, and there is no evidence that the elementary bodies belonging to this kingdom are capable of producing any form of fever; and because there is indubitable evidence that organic matter in a recent state of putrescence—the more recent the more potent—is capable of producing the most deadly forms of fever. From these considerations it is conjectured that the primary cause, whatever it be, is some subtle fluid which has not wholly lost its organic composition, and that it consists of particles of extreme minuteness, capable of attaching itself to the surfaces of other bodies, and even of increasing under favourable circumstances.

It is further thought that this body is not equally diffused through the atmosphere, but is only partially distributed, and that this accounts for the local distribution of epidemics, and for their occasional absence from places which apparently present all the conditions favourable to their development.

Lastly, the opinion is gaining ground, that this body acts in the manner of a ferment. It is urged in favour of this view, that a ferment being an azotized substance in a state of putrefactive alteration, the body in question must find, in the decomposing organic compounds with which impure blood is charged, precisely the materials for taking on the fermenting process. The advocates for this view think that the term "*zymotic*" is not only the appropriate name of the whole of this class of diseases, but that it also declares an interesting fact connected with them. Whatever may be the truth with respect to these points, on which at present we have no positive knowledge, one thing is certain, that practically our concern is with the known causes,—the ascertained conditions. These are palpable, definite, and capable of complete removal and prevention.

Overcrowding, for example, we can prevent; the accumulation of filth in towns and houses we can prevent; the supply of light, air, and water, together with the several other appliances included in the all-comprehensive word CLEANLINESS, we can secure. To the extent to which it is in our power to do this, it is in our power to prevent epidemics.

The human family have now lived together in communities more than six thousand years, yet they have not learnt to make their habitations clean. At last we are beginning to learn the lesson. When we shall have mastered it, we shall have conquered epidemics. Our duties, then, and our hopes in this respect, I shall proceed to show.

***

The principal constituents of the atmosphere maintain their equilibrium steadily over the whole surface of the globe. There is scarcely any difference in the relative proportion of its oxygen and nitrogen in the torrid zone and in the arctic regions. Whatever influence the atmosphere may have on climate must consequently depend on something adventitious to it and not in anything forming a part of it. Possibly therefore that something may be, in some degree, under human control.

The main constituents of climate are temperature and moisture, and these are the climatic conditions that exercise the greatest influence on epidemics.

Minor but still important conditions are the nature of the soil, the proportion of land that is cleared and under cultivation, the extent of forests, lakes, and rivers, the prevailing winds, the electrical state of the atmosphere, and so on.

The temperature is highest where the sun's rays are vertical, or nearly so; where the sky is cloudless; where the day is longest; and where there is the smallest difference between the fervid noon-tide heat and the temperature of the short night.

The moisture is greatest where in addition to all the other sources of humidity there are periodical rains. In the countries subject to these rains, the entire extent of the level and low land is often covered a foot deeper with water than before the rain set in.

Elevated temperature and excessive moisture are combined in tropical countries; and they are concentrated in those parts of the tropics in which there are extensive forests having an undergrowth of luxuriant vegetation; in which the tides of the ocean penetrate deeply into the interior of the land, and mix with the waters of the rivers; and in which the rivers constantly overflow their banks and form marshes and swamps.

In tropical countries there are tracts such as these that extend in unbroken continuity hundreds of leagues. The western coast of Africa (the Bight of Benin) presents an unbroken area of upwards of 100,000 square miles, consisting of one vast alluvial and densely-wooded forest, irrigated by Atlantic tides, and intersected by numerous rivers and creeks, whose muddy banks are constantly overflowed.

In describing a tropical forest, Humboldt says, "Under the bushy, deep, green verdure of trees of stupendous height and size, there reigns constantly a kind of half daylight, a sort of obscurity, of which our forests of pines, oaks, and beech trees afford no example; forming a carpet of verdure, the dark tint of which augments the splendour of the aërial light."

With this luxuriance of vegetation is combined a corresponding abundance of animal life. The earth and air teem with living creatures.

"The mould," observes the same distinguished traveller, "contains the spoils of innumerable quantities of reptiles, worms, and insects. Wherever the soil is turned up we are struck with a mass of organic substances, which by turns are developed, transformed, and decomposed. Nature in these climates appear more active, more fruitful, we might say more prodigal of life."

The air is still more alive than the land. Insects fill the lower strata of the atmosphere to the height of fifteen or twenty feet, like a condensed vapour. It is estimated that a cubic foot of air is often peopled by a million of winged insects, which contain a caustic and venomous liquid, several species being nearly two lines (1.8) long.

When two persons who have their home in these regions meet in the morning, the first questions they address to each other are, "How did you find the zancudoes during the night?" "How are we to-day for the mosquitoes?" An ancient form of Chinese politeness, showing the ancient state of that country, was—"Have you been incommoded in the night by serpents?"

It appears that there are still inhabited places in which the Chinese compliment on the serpents might be added to that of the mosquitoes.

Proportionate to this prodigality of organic life is the amount of organic decomposition, the products of which are poured into the atmosphere and suspended in the surrounding vapour and fog,[11] to which they give a decided and often a highly offensive odour.

11. See note, p. 16.

"On fixing our eyes on the tops of the trees," describes Humboldt, "we discovered streams of vapour wherever a solar ray penetrated and traversed the dense atmosphere, exhaling, together with the aromatic odour yielded by the flowers, the fruit, and even the wood, that peculiar odour which we perceive in autumn in foggy seasons. It might be said, that notwithstanding the elevated temperature the air cannot dissolve the quantity of water exhaled from the surface of the soil and of the vegetation."

"At the distance of several miles from the coast," says Dr Daniell, in describing the western shores of Africa, "the peculiar odour arising from swampy exhalations and the decomposition of vegetable matter is very perceptible, and sometimes even offensive. The water also is frequently of a dusky hue, with leaves, branches, and other vegetable debris floating on the surface, brought down from the interior by innumerable narrow channels that empty their turbid streams into the open ocean."

It is under these climatic conditions that the worst forms of epidemics are engendered: the most sudden in their attack, the most rapid in their development, the most general in their prevalence, and the most mortal.

The form of the epidemic prevalent in any particular district is dependent on the physical characters of the immediate neighbourhood. Thus intermittents prevail chiefly in marshy and swampy districts: remittents also chiefly there, though not exclusively; while in other localities other forms arise approximating to the continued type of temperate climates.

For the most part these epidemics are strictly endemic, and are confined to the particular regions in which they are engendered. They never pass the limit of the equatorial or tropical zone. Yellow Fever, one of the most common and destructive of these diseases, is still more restricted in its range, being confined within a definite line determined by temperature. It is incapable of existing where the average range of the thermometer is greater than from 76° to 86° of Fahrenheit, or where the temperature varies more than from 5° to 10° night and day. Extreme heat and moderate cold immediately stop it; nay, even the prevalence of a cold wind for a few hours only.

In other instances these epidemics pass beyond the regions in which they are produced, and sometimes extend to all the other quarters of the globe. The Black Death, the range of which we have seen, was engendered in China; the Cholera of our own day, generated in the delta of the Ganges, the great source and centre of Indian epidemics, ravaged that country long before it directed its course to Europe.

When these tropical epidemics advance into more temperate climes, they lay aside nothing of their nature; they lose but little of their power. Wherever they go they decimate the populations which they attack.

One remarkable peculiarity of some of these epidemics is, that natives of the region in which they prevail are for the most part unsusceptible to them. This is true however only of particular forms of pestilence. Some of them acknowledge no acclimation. Cholera, for example, attacks equally natives and new comers. On the other hand, yellow fever rarely attacks the natives who reside permanently within its zone. Its chief victims are strangers who have recently arrived within its sphere, particularly the inhabitants of northern climates. The susceptibility to its influence appears to be strictly proportionate to the degree of northern latitude from which the stranger has arrived, and the shortness of the interval that has passed since he left the European for the Equatorial regions.

We see something of the same kind in the wide-spread epidemics of our own country. During the prevalence of Cholera it was observed over and over again, that persons coming directly from the pure air of the country into the infected part of a town, were seized with the disease. The explanation is not obvious. It would seem, however, to be connected with the suddenness of the shock on the system. Priestley found, that after shutting up a mouse in a given quantity of air a considerable time, it seemed to be weak, and to be slowly dying. If at this period he put a fresh mouse into the same air, it instantly died. It seems as if the system can bear a pestiferous atmosphere better when gradually than when suddenly exposed to it.

I do not know that I can give a more vivid picture of a tropical epidemic than that which is afforded by the outbreak of Cholera in the 86th regiment at Kurrachee in June, 1846.

On this occasion the atmosphere was very peculiar,—damp, hot, stagnant, and oppressive. Not a breath of air was stirring. A few isolated cases of cholera had occurred for some days. The utmost alarm was excited in the minds of experienced persons, who felt certain that an epidemic was at hand. Their fears were too fully realized. On the night of the 15th, upwards of 40 men were seized with cholera in its severest form; in two days more 256 were attacked, of whom 131 were already dead.

"The floors of the hospital," says Dr Thom, the surgeon of the regiment, "were literally strewed with the livid bodies of men labouring under the pangs of premature dissolution. Many were brought in with the cold and clammy damp of death; as if sudden obstruction of every vital function had taken place, and the fountains of life had been arrested by an invisible but instantaneous shock. It was indeed a sight never to be forgotten, to behold the powerful frames of the finest men of a fine corps, who had that morning been in apparent good health, and most of them on the evening parade, as if at once stricken down, and striving, with the last efforts of gigantic strength, to resist a death-call that would not be refused."

In describing a river on the west coast of Africa, Dr Daniell says— "When I visited it, I found two vessels moored a short distance from its mouth, one of which within the space of five months had buried two entire crews, a solitary person alone surviving. The other, which had arrived at a much later period, had been similarly deprived of one-half of its men, and the remainder were in such a debilitated condition as to be incapable of undertaking any active or laborious duty. Immediately before, another vessel had sailed from this port in such a deplorable state as to be solely dependent on the aid of Kroomen to perform the voyage."

In the statistical report of Sir Alexander Tulloch it is stated, that out of 1658 white troops sent out to military stations on the western coast of Africa, 1271 perished from climatic diseases; while of the 387 who remained to be sent home, 17 died on their passage; 157 were reported as incapable of further service; and 180 as qualified only for garrison service; thus leaving only 33 out of 1658 men who were fit for active service.

As we pass out of the torrid zone a remarkable change takes place in the general character of epidemics. They lose more and more of their intermittent type, and become either remittent or continued. The remittent keeps its hold over the southern part of Europe, and continually breaks out in the form of Yellow Fever. As we proceed northward out of the yellow fever zone, that disease wholly disappears, and typhus and its kindred maladies take its place; typhus commencing precisely at the point where yellow fever ends.

There is, indeed, one of the ordinary diseases of temperate climes, and only one, which appears capable of penetrating within the torrid zone, and of committing greater ravages there than in lower temperatures, and that is Small-pox. With this exception, the ordinary epidemics of temperate climates do not enter the tropics, while, on the other hand, the ordinary epidemics of the tropics every now and then decimate the temperate regions.

"In these our latitudes," says Dr William Fergusson, "cold and fatigue, and sorrow and hunger, will generate fever anywhere; but every region, every climate, will exhibit its own form of fever. With us it is Typhus; in the warmer countries of Europe, Remittent; in the upper Mediterranean, Plague; in the Antilles and Western Africa, Yellow Fever; this last being restricted to particular localities, temperatures, and elevation. While typhus fever goes out when you enter the tropics, it is there that yellow fever commences; the pure epidemic of a hot climate that cannot be transported or communicated upon any other ground. Places, not persons, constitute the rule of its existence. Places, not persons, comprehend the whole history, the etiology of the disease. Places, not persons! Let the emphatic words be dinned into the ears of the Lords of the Treasury, of Trade and Plantations, until they acquire the force of a creed, which will save them hereafter from the absurdity of enforcing a quarantine[12] in England against an amount of solar heat of which its climate is insusceptible. Let them further be repeated in the Schools of Medicine until the Professors become ashamed of imbuing the minds of the young with prejudice and false belief, which, should they ever visit warmer climates, may cause them to be eminently mischievous in vexing the commerce and deeply and injuriously agitating the public mind of whatever community may have received them."

<u>12</u>. See Cases of the Eclair, Dygden, &c., *post.*

Climate differs not only in different countries but in different parts of the same country. The climate of the country is different from that of the city. The climate of every city, town, and village, differs from that of every other. The temperature, the moisture, and the other meteorological conditions of different districts, nay, even of different streets in the same town, vary to such a degree as to influence materially their relative salubrity and the prevalence or absence of particular classes of disease. These local climatic conditions and their connection with prevalent diseases, have not as yet received due attention: when they shall have received it—and they will receive it—a new light will be shed on local epidemics.

***

I pass now to CIVILIZATION.

We have no sufficient knowledge of the state of the people and of their diseases, in any of the civilized nations of antiquity, to trace the relation between them. The authentic history of periods, comparatively near to our own time, as far as concerns the diseases of the people, goes scarcely further back than the 14th century. The first great epidemic, to which I have so often called attention, occurred in that century, and we have reliable evidence, both of the phenomena attending this plague and the condition of the people at that time. I assume this period therefore as my starting-point.

I take a civilized community to be one in which there exist—

1. A sovereign authority.

2. Laws incorruptibly administered.

3. Physical comfort generally diffused.

4. Intellectual development and activity generally diffused.

5. Recognition of the fundamental principles of religion and morality.

Without the two first, there can be no security for life and property, both of which must be placed in absolute and unquestionable safety before a single step can be taken out of the lowest depth of barbarism. Without the two last, none of the others can be acquired. These conditions are therefore the basis of the pyramid of society.

Taking these then as the essential constituents of civilization, and applying them as a test to Great Britain, we shall see that at the commencement of the 14th century England was in a state of barbarism, since every one of these elements was wanting, although the foundation of political and social institutions containing the germs of liberty and progress had been already laid.

Practically, however, at that period there was no sovereign authority, for the king had no sufficient power to maintain order, to protect the rights and liberties of the people, or to defend his own throne against armed men nominally his subjects; while the lord of every feudal castle exercised a more perfect sovereignty over his vassals than the so-called monarch over the nation.

Every town was a fortress, and every house in which it was safe to dwell a castle, the inmates of which, like people in a garrison, constantly held themselves prepared to resist attack, from which they were never secure. They slept with arms at their side.

Marauders openly encamped on the public roads for the plunder of the wayfarer, which often ended in his murder. Few persons ventured to travel alone, and none without the reasonable apprehension that they might never return alive.

Scarcely a third part of the area of the kingdom was under cultivation. The remainder consisted of moor, forest, and fen. Vast tracts were under water during the greater part of the year, and at other times formed morasses, marshes, and swamps.

Immediately beyond the walls that encompassed the towns were large stagnant ditches, which being the nearest receptacles for refuse, were full of all sorts of decomposing filth.

The streets were narrow, unpaved, undrained, uncleansed, and unlighted. There was no provision for the removal of the town refuse. Gutters were formed at the sides of the streets, as in Bethnal Green and the neglected parts of all our towns at the present time, into which the inhabitants threw the refuse of their houses; forming in dry weather a semi-fluid mass of corrupting animal and vegetable matter, and in rainy weather black turbid rivulets which ultimately poured their contents into some water-course.

The houses were mean and squalid, built of wood and wattles, thatched with straw, without chimneys, the windows without glass, the floors without boards, the furniture of the rudest description; the use of linen was scarcely known; common straw formed the king's bed. "The floors," says

Erasmus, writing two centuries later, "generally are made of nothing but loam, and are strewed with rushes, which being constantly put on fresh, without a removal of the old, remain lying there, in some cases for twenty years; with fish bones, broken victuals, the dregs of tankards, and impregnated with other filth underneath, from dogs and men." Contemporary writers concur in representing the offensive odour of decaying straw and rushes as universal in the houses.

There was no knowledge of the art of collecting, preserving, and storing fodder. The animals for winter food were slaughtered in autumn, and their flesh salted or smoked. It was only during three months of the year, from Midsummer to Michaelmas, that any fresh animal food, excepting game and river fish, was tasted even by the nobles of the land. The common people subsisted chiefly on salted beef, veal, and pork, the price of which was one-half less than that of wheat in the time of Henry VIII.

There were no fresh vegetables. As late as the 18th century salads were sent from Holland for the table of Queen Caroline. Sir John Pringle, writing in the middle of the last century, states that his father's gardener told him that in the time of his grandfather cabbages were sold for a crown a-piece. It was not until towards the close of the 16th century (1585) that the potato was first brought to England, where it was limited to the garden for at least a century and a half after it had been planted by Sir Walter Raleigh in his own garden. It was first cultivated as a field crop in Scotland so recently as the year 1752.

For many centuries England remained in the condition of country in which no more subsistence is produced than is barely sufficient for the necessities of the people. Consequently every year of scarcity became a year of famine, and such years, about one in ten, occurred for ages with great regularity, and often equalled in their terrible results the worst famines of antiquity.

In a cold climate fuel is nearly as important as food, for which indeed it is a substitute. A large portion of our daily food is used up in supporting that internal fire by which the heat of the human body in every climate, and under every variety of external temperature, is maintained at the 98th degree of Fahrenheit. The greater the loss of heat by cooling, the greater the amount of heat which the body itself must generate to maintain its temperature at this elevated point. This demand for additional heat cannot be supplied without additional quantities of food, and unless these supplies are afforded, the substance of the body itself, its very tissues and organs, are consumed; a process which cannot be continued long without exhaustion, disease, and death. The phrase "starved by cold" expresses a more literal fact than is commonly understood. Unhappily the circumstances which deprive a population of the means of counteracting cold limit also the supplies of food at their command, and the pressure of the twofold privation, want of food and want of fuel, commonly occurs at the very season when both these indispensable supports of life are most needed. Some conception may be formed of the suffering to which our ancestors were exposed from this cause, from the fact that their prejudice against the use of coal as an article of fuel was such that a law was passed rendering it a capital offence to burn it within the City, and there is a record in the Tower importing that a person was tried, convicted, and executed for this offence in the reign of Edward the First. It was not until the reign of Charles the First that there was a regular supply of coals to London.

The habits of the people increased the force of these privations. Intemperance was a national vice. Excessive carousing at home, or days and nights spent in taverns, was the usual practice among all classes, and the physical and moral evils resulting from the custom were neither redeemed nor lessened by the epithet which these habitual convivialities appear to have conferred upon the nation of "Merrie England." Caius, indeed, one of the most celebrated physicians of the sixteenth century, couples Germany and the Netherlands with England in this common reproach. "These three nations," he says, "destroy more meats and drynkes without all order, convenient time, reason, and necessitie, than all other countries under the son, to the great annoyance of their bodies and wittes."

This condition of the country and this mode of life themselves constitute the most powerful causes of epidemics; and an extraordinary concurrence and concentration of these causes are manifested in the combination of the circumstances which have been enumerated, namely, in the malarious state of the greater part of the kingdom, in the confined space of the towns, in the deficiency and putrescency of the food, in the inadequacy of the means of protection from cold, and in the intemperance of the people. These were the true sources of the malignity and mortality of the pestilences of that age.

We have no reliable evidence of the actual mortality produced by these terrible diseases; for no physician has left such an account of the epidemics of which he was an eye-witness as enables us to determine it, and there was no Registrar-General to fill up the momentous columns included in his death-roll. We can therefore only take the statements of the time as we find them.

According to the accounts of contemporary writers, the Black Death swept away, within the space of four years, a fourth part of the population of Europe. Some towns in England are stated to have lost two-thirds of their inhabitants, and it is computed that one-half of the entire population of the country perished.

Of the Sweating Sickness, Bacon says it "destroyed infinite persons;" Stowe "a wonderful number;" and other writers reckon the deaths in the places attacked by thousands.

Similar representations are given of the ravages of the Plague, of the Petechial Fever, and even occasionally of Intermittent Fever; and the substantial correctness of these statements is confirmed by entries in parish registers still extant, which tell the story of the local outbreaks of those days with graphic and touching simplicity.

During some of the worst of these visitations, contemporary writers concur in stating that the living were insufficient to bury the dead; business was suspended; the courts of law were closed; the churches were deserted for want of a sufficient number of clergy to perform the service; and ships were seen driving about on the ocean and drifting on shore, whose crews had perished to the last man.

We can form no adequate conception of the terror inspired by these events. We have seen alarm in our own day, but then it bordered on maniacal despair. It seemed as if the last judgment had come upon the world, and men abandoned alike their possessions and their friends. The rich gave up their treasures and laid them at the foot of the altars; neighbour abandoned neighbour; parents their offspring, and brothers their sisters. "If" says one of the chroniclers, "in a circle of friends any one only by a single word happened to bring the plague to mind, first one and then another of the company was seized with a tormenting anguish; certain that they were attacked with a mortal sickness, they slunk away home, and there soon yielded up the ghost."

These fearful forms of pestilence were accompanied by moral epidemics more appalling than the physical. Of these the two following may serve as examples:—

Vast assemblages of men and women formed circles hand in hand, dancing, leaping, shouting, insensible to external impressions; some seeing visions and spirits whose names they shrieked out; others in epileptic convulsions with foaming at the mouth; all continuing to make the most violent muscular exertions for hours together, until they fell to the ground in a state of exhaustion. Lookers-on were seized with an uncontrollable impulse to join in these wild revels. Peasants left their ploughs, mechanics their workshops, servants their masters, boys and girls their parents, women their domestic duties, and men their business, thus to spend days and nights; these infatuated crowds passing furiously through streets, along highways, over fields, and from town to town. This madness pervaded the least barbarous countries of Europe for upwards of two centuries, under the name of the "Dancing Mania." It was universally attributed to demoniacal possession, and its cure was attempted by exorcism. It was one expression and outlet of the violent passions of that time, imposture and profligacy playing principal parts in this strange drama.

More pernicious than this madness was the mania of cruelty, an especial manifestation of which was the ferocious persecution of the Jews, who were put to death by hundreds and thousands, under the accusation that they had poisoned the wells. At Basle a number of this nation, whose European history proves them to have been everywhere amongst the most inoffensive of the people, were enclosed in a wooden building and burnt with it. At Strasburg two thousand were burnt alive. Whoever showed them compassion and endeavoured to protect them were put upon the rack and burnt with them. In numerous instances these unhappy people, driven to despair, assembled in their own habitations, to which they set fire and consumed themselves with their families. The noble and the mean bound themselves by an oath to extirpate them from the face of the earth by fire and sword.

In England this relentless cruelty took particularly the shape of burning innocent people under the name of witches; an infatuation which pervaded all classes from the highest to the lowest, affording a melancholy exemplification of the close alliance between credulity and cruelty.[13]

13. The number of wretched beings condemned and executed for this imaginary crime at the Assizes of Suffolk and Essex alone, in the year 1646, amounted to two hundred. Dr Zachary Gray affirms that he had seen an authentic account of persons who had so suffered in the whole of England, amounting to from three to four thousand. So late as the year 1697 seven persons, three men and four women, were burnt at Paisley for this alleged crime. We seldom sufficiently consider how near we are to those times of dreadful superstition and cruelty! How short a period it is since the light of a brighter day dawned upon us!

But in the midst of these terrible disorders, changes which had been in silent operation during several centuries began to produce visible results. The independent power of the nobles had been suppressed; the feuds that raged between them, filling the country with disorder and bloodshed, had been put down; the supremacy of the law had been established; property and life had become more secure; industry had taken a surprising start; the practical abolition of serfdom had been to a large extent effected; and at last came the final breaking up of the feudal system in the reign of Henry VII. by the passing of the law authorizing the alienation of land.

About the middle of the fifteenth century improvements in the condition of the people, which had been gradually effected by these changes, were accelerated by a succession of events that gave an extraordinary impulse to the human mind, just aroused from the long and deep sleep of the middle ages—that dark night which was now passing away.

Among the most memorable of these was the invention of printing, which the three immortal masters of the art had now completed (1436–1442), giving untiring and undying wings to thought;—

The diffusion over the West of Europe of the remains of a former civilization, by the dispersion of the treasures of classical art, literature, and science, which before Constantinople fell into the hands of barbarians (1453) had been confined within the walls of that city;—

The cessation of the long and disastrous struggle between the East and the West, by the expulsion of the Moors from Spain (1492);—

The discovery of the New World;—

And lastly, the Reformation, that stupendous work which with giant strength burst asunder the chain which consummate skill and supreme power had spent ages in forging and riveting: that stupendous work, which was not merely emancipation from spiritual bondage, but the re-communication of the long-lost spirit of religion; the noble men who achieved it being ever, even in their day of triumph, less intent on demolishing the gorgeous edifice that had held the mind enthralled, than on erecting a pure temple in which it might worship with sincerity and freedom.

The time when the foundation was laid for this intellectual and spiritual renovation was also that of the commencement of physical improvement. The towns being no longer fortresses, it became unnecessary to maintain their fortifications. Walls were thrown down; stagnant moats were filled up; broader streets were opened; more convenient houses were erected. Forests were cleared; marshes and swamps were drained; more land was brought under cultivation; more vegetable matter was produced; the art of collecting, storing, and preserving fodder was discovered. Fresh meat became the food of the people during a longer period of the year; in the course of two centuries the length of that period had doubled, and at last such food was in use the whole winter. The products of growing art and manufacture superseded the beds of straw and displaced the floors of rushes. Famines ceased. There has been no recurrence of famine in England since the middle of the 15th century (1448). The proportion of people in the enjoyment of moderate competence rapidly increased. It is computed that in the 16th century the number of small freeholders realizing a clear income of between £60 and £70 a-year amounted with their families to one-seventh of the whole population, and that the number of persons who tilled their own land was greater than the number of those who farmed the land of others.[14]

<u>14</u>. Macaulay's History, Vol. I. Chap. III.

In the next century the care of the Public Health became a recognized and direct object of the Legislature and the Magistracy. Better regulations were enforced in the metropolis for the removal of filth, for the construction and extension of sewers, and for widening, paving, and lighting the streets. In the middle of this century the Great Fire (1666) consumed 13,000 houses and left an open space of upwards of a square mile. This opportunity of improvement was not lost. Though in rebuilding the city the same lines of streets were preserved, and the streets were still kept much too narrow, yet there was some improvement in the general plan, while the houses were built of better materials; brick was substituted for wood and plaster, and the buildings were less crowded and less projecting.

The spirit of improvement thus awakened exerted itself with increased effect during the whole of the eighteenth century. Agriculture, which was now rapidly advancing, had created a demand for town refuse, the fertilizing property of which began to be perceived; so that all manner of offensive substances were regularly carried away to the fields, to the great increase of the cleanliness of the streets. At the same time many of the narrower streets were widened, the houses were entirely taken down and rebuilt, and in this operation slate was universally substituted for thatch, and brick for timber. The pavement also, which had long been the reproach of London, was improved. Population in the mean time rapidly increased, less by the relative increase of the number of births than by the proportionate decrease of the deaths, and this notwithstanding the occasional occurrence of severe pestilence. The result of the whole was an increase in the length of life.

An increase in the length of life is an expression and a measure of the sum of comfort experienced from the whole collective circumstances that make up national prosperity. In the interval between the seventeenth and eighteenth centuries that sum grew into a highly important one. Of this the proof is positive.

It happened that in the year 1693 a loan was raised for the service of the State by the method of Tontine, and that another was contracted by the same method in the year 1790; the interval being almost exactly a century.

The term Tontine is derived from the name of the originator of this scheme of life annuity, the principle of which is this. The person who advances £100 is at liberty to name any life he pleases, during the existence of which he draws a certain annuity; and as the shares of the dead nominees are distributed among the living ones, the annuity continually increases till the last survivor gets the whole income.

A comparison of the experience between two Tontines gives the exact measure of the effect produced on the duration of life, by such changes in the social condition of the people as may have occurred in the interval between them.

A person of the male sex (for there is a considerable difference in the results in the two sexes), living in 1793, compared with a male living in 1690, at fifteen years of age, had gained an expectation of life of nearly ten years; at twenty years of age, nine years and a half; at twenty-five years of age, upwards of eight years; at thirty years of age, upwards of seven years, and so on.

Or the gain in the expectation of life may be stated more correctly in years, thus: Take for example a man at the age of 30, in 1693 his expectation of life would have been 26.665; in 1790 it would have been 33.775 years.

On this evidence Mr Finlaison justly observes that civilization could not have increased by a single leap in the time of Mr Pitt, but must have been slowly on the increase at least since the days of Queen Anne.

We may then fairly conclude, that in the interval between the close of the 17th and 18th centuries human life gained an addition equivalent to a fourth part of its whole term. What has it gained in the succeeding century? What has been the increase in the value of life in this first half of the century in which we ourselves have lived? Though unfortunately we can appeal to the results of no renewed tontine to enable us to answer this question with exactness,[15] yet there are not wanting evidences that the value of life continues progressively to increase. It must necessarily continue to increase, because the main conditions on which life and health depend have experienced, during the whole of the present century, an expansion and improvement, on which no former age presents a parallel. It will be sufficient to establish this fact, to glance at what has been effected within this period in the multiplication and diffusion of the three primary necessaries of existence—food, clothing, and fuel.

Such has been the increased production of food during the present century, that the quantity now raised maintains ten millions more human beings than existed at its commencement; for on the first enumeration of the people in 1801 the population of Great Britain was eleven millions; in 1851, it was twenty-one millions.[16]

15. Considering that there appears to be no objection in principle to the method of raising a loan by Tontine, and that the scheme is a popular one, it seems highly desirable that we should continue this means of measuring with positive exactness the results of our advancing civilization.

16. According to Mr Rickman, from the best information that can be obtained from Doomsday Book, the population of England in the time of William the Conqueror was 1½ millions.

In the reign of Edward the Third (1377), when a poll-tax was imposed on all persons of both sexes above fourteen, it was 2½ millions.

In the reign of Queen Elizabeth, at the period of the Spanish Armada, it was 4 millions.

According to Mr Finlaison, at the close of the 16th century it was somewhat under 5 millions two hundred thousand.

According to Mr Rickman, on a computation founded on the return of Baptisms, as stated in the Abstract of Parish Registers, it was in 1700, 5½ millions; in 1750, 6½ millions; and in 1770, 7½ millions.

The first actual enumeration was made in 1801. The following table exhibits the rate of increase in the population of Great Britain from that time up to the enumeration in 1851:

YEARS.	POPULATION.	INCREASE Each Decennial Period.	ANNUAL RATE of Increase per cent.
1801	10,917,433		
1811	12,424,120	1,506,687	1.274
1821	14,402,643	1,978,523	1.489
1831	16,564,138	2,161,495	1.408
1841	18,813,786	2,249,648	1.279
1851	21,121,967	2,308,181	1.186

This increased production of food consists chiefly of grain, green crops, and garden vegetables, countless in variety, and highly nutritious and grateful, completely reversing the nature of the national subsistence compared with that of former times, and giving to the masses of the people a constant and unfailing supply, winter and summer, of fresh vegetable nutriment.

This increased production of food is mainly of home growth, for the supply of wheat from foreign sources would scarcely suffice to afford to each person two gallons of flour annually.

This increased production has been obtained partly by a progressive increase in the quantity of land brought under cultivation, which now amounts for the United Kingdom to upwards of 40,000,000 of acres, by far the greater part of which is employed in the production of human food; and partly by the employment of capital in the improvement of the soil, by which large tracts that a few years ago were wholly sterile, or deemed incapable of producing wheat, now yield some of the finest grain in England.[17]

> 17. "In 1821 almost the only grain produced in the Fens of Cambridgeshire consisted of oats; since then, by draining and manuring, the capability of the soil has been so changed that these fens now produce some of the finest wheat that is grown in England; and this more costly grain now constitutes the main dependence of the farmers in a district where 14 years ago its produce was scarcely attempted."—*Porter's Progress of the Nation.*

This increased fertility of the soil renders it more healthy by diminishing its moisture and raising its temperature. One cubic foot of water in the process of evaporation deprives three millions of cubic feet of air of one degree of temperature. An undrained field growing rushes has a permanent temperature from four to six degrees lower than an adjoining field drained and growing wheat. By draining and manuring, by throwing down fences, by removing trees, by clearing underwood, and by promoting the free aëration of the soil, the temperature of large tracts of land in the north of England has been permanently raised three degrees. Thus that very culture of the earth, by which it is made to yield the largest amount of food, increases its salubrity as an abode for man, and lessens at their source the main causes of epidemics.

This increased production has been obtained by a proportionally small addition to labour; for while the quantity of land brought under cultivation, and its produce, have been increasing at a rate of which there is no similar example in any age or country, the relative number of persons employed in agriculture has been as steadily decreasing. As long as the labour of a man applied to the cultivation of the soil is capable of producing only a bare subsistence for himself, there can be no advance in civilization. But when two men can produce subsistence for three, the labour of the third can be set free for the production of surplus articles, which add to the sum of the general convenience, and from that moment the community takes a start in the career of improvement. From a comparison of occupations taken in 1831, it appears that, at that time, the division of labour among the people was such that one person raised nearly all the food of home production consumed by four persons.[18]

18. Porter's Progress of the Nation, Chap. III.

Were the remaining three idle? Mediately or immediately they were engaged in producing clothing, or fuel, or machinery, economizing the production of both; and busily and well they worked.

In number they exceed one million and a half. Taking into account the accessory occupations, indeed, no fewer than one million two hundred thousand are employed on one single material alone, namely cotton. For these workers, at the beginning of the century, there were imported yearly 56 millions of pounds of cotton: at present the annual importation of it exceeds 550 millions of pounds. These workers in 1820 were assisted in their operations by fourteen thousand power-looms; at present they are assisted by three hundred thousand power-looms, besides twenty-five millions of spindles;[19] while each power-loom, superintended by an adult assisted by a child, completes weekly twenty times the amount of work which the hand-loom is capable of producing. The increase of production is of course enormous, and the effect is a progressive cheapening of the articles manufactured, reducing the price of some of them tenfold, and placing them within the reach of the poorest classes:[20] articles of clothing not only conducive to health through warmth, but almost equally so through cleanliness; for they are almost all composed of such tissues and textures as favour and compel frequent washing.

19. Return to the House of Commons by the Factory Inspectors, of the Number of Cotton, Woollen, Worsted, Flax, and Silk Factories subject to the Factories Acts in the United Kingdom, page 21.

20. The cheapness of some of these ornamental as well as useful fabrics is calculated to excite astonishment. A yard of platt net is worth from 20s. to £5; a yard of plain net may be bought for one shilling.

Gigantic strides have been made at the same time in another article of clothing, the basis of which is wool, and of which there were imported in 1801 seven millions of pounds; in 1844, sixty-three millions of pounds. This enormous importation of foreign wool has not only not diminished its home growth, but the increased demand for it has led to a vast multiplication of the animals that yield it, and what is of equal importance, has induced an extraordinary care in improving their breed; so that the very means which have fed the steam-engine have fed the people both with more plentiful and with better food; the steam-engine, meanwhile, applied to these and to all manufacturing processes, being as much a producer of food as the plough.[21]

21. Similar progress has been made in the manufacture of flax and silk as of cotton and wool.

And the same is emphatically true of fuel, the main creator of all this activity and of its astonishing results; this necessary of life being now brought to the door of every family in three-fold abundance and at one-half the price at which it could have been obtained at the commencement of the century; while such is the demand for it in various manufactures of vast magnitude, that one trade alone, that of iron, consumes annually eight millions of tons—a trade which immediately and powerfully facilitates the production both of food and of clothing. Thus, like one of Nature's beautiful adaptations, like that wonderful cycle, for example, in which production, change, and reproduction go on in an unvarying circle, the constant and abundant supply of one main necessary of life furnishes the means of producing the others; while these last are the immediate causes of the abundance of the first.

And what a busy hive does this country present at the present time! Out of every thousand males twenty years of age in the kingdom, 836 are directly employed in some active occupation contributing to the national wealth; while the remaining 114 are by no means idle, for they are engaged in some one of the professions.

Though the masses have not yet obtained their due share of the wealth they create, and though there is a class which in relation to one essential condition, to be stated immediately, civilization has scarcely reached, or reached only to injure—with these exceptions, no doubt very important ones—the evidence is indubitable that the entire body of society, from its base to its apex, stands on an elevated table-land which many centuries have been employed in raising and consolidating. I have partly proved this by showing the general diffusion of the means of healthful subsistence and the prolongation of life. I am now to prove it by applying these facts to the subject more especially before us, the decline and disappearance of epidemics.

It is now exactly two centuries, short of ten years, since the visitation of the Great Plague of 1665—that terrible disease which ravaged England for the space of 1249 years: for it is first heard of in English history in the year 430, and the last year in which its name appears in the Bills of Mortality is 1679; that terrible disease which not only maintained undiminished power over this vast space of time, but which sometimes recurred twenty times in one century—that terrible disease is gone. It cannot be supposed that it has worn itself out, for it still frequently returns with its ancient malignity to Constantinople, Alexandria, Smyrna, and other Eastern States.

Petechial or Jail fever, the fatal scourge of the ship, the prison, the hospital, the school, and in short of every place in which any considerable number of persons was assembled, and which when it once broke out was as destructive as the plague—that terrible disease is gone.

Intermittent fever, which in the middle of the fifteenth century and long afterwards recurred like the plague periodically but more frequently, and which often raged as universally, which was sometimes so mortal that the living could hardly bury the dead, and which spared not even the throne, for James I. and Oliver Cromwell both died of ague contracted in London—that formidable disease is gone. Ague, it is true, still exists in the fenny and marshy places which yet remain in England, and we occasionally see a case contracted there in the wards of the London Fever Hospital, but I have not seen a single case of ague contracted in London for upwards of a quarter of a century.

Remittent fever is also gone, scurvy is gone, rickets is gone, malignant sore throat is gone, typhus-gravior is gone, and if small-pox is not gone it is entirely the consequence of our own apathy and folly.

No less remarkable is the gradual decline and the ultimate cessation of certain forms of bowel-complaint of a very painful nature, the very names of which have long disappeared both from medical and popular language. In the 17th century the deaths from two of these diseases alone registered in the Bills of Mortality under two separate titles, were never less than 1000 annually, and in some years they exceeded 4000; but from having been 1070 in the year 1700, they decreased through each successive decade of that century in the following remarkable progression: 770, 706, 350, 150, 110, 80, 70, 40, 20; and they have so entirely disappeared during the 19th century, that, as I have just said, their very names are no longer in use.

Moreover several acute diseases which hardly come under the name of Epidemics, such as Rheumatic Fever, Pneumonia, and Peripneumonia, are much less frequent and fatal now than they were a century ago.

All this time there has been a continually decreasing mortality. In 1700 the estimated mortality of England and Wales was 1 in 39; in 1750 it was 1 in 40; in 1801 it was 1 in 44; in 1810 it was 1 in 49; in 1820 it was 1 in 55, and in 1830 it was 1 in 58.

In London in 1700[22] the deaths were 1 in 25; in 1750, 1 in 21;[23] in 1801, 1 in 35; in 1810, 1 in 38; and in 1830, 1 in 45.

22. parliamentary Returns, 1811.

23. It is conceived that the remarkable increase of the mortality in the middle of this century was mainly caused by the abuse of spirituous liquors, which was checked about that time by the imposition of high duties.—*Sir Gilbert Blane's Dissertations.*

The diminishing number of those who are born merely to die exhibits the decrease of mortality in a still more striking point of view. The estimated mortality of persons under twenty years of age in London in 1780 was 1 in 76; in 1801 it was 1 in 96; in 1830 it was 1 in 124; in 1833 it was 1 in 137; not much more than one-half the proportion who died under twenty half a century ago.

The contrast between the mortality of former times and of the present is seen in the mortality of London in 1685 and in 1830. In the first period the deaths were 1 in 23; in the second they were 1 in 45, little more than one-half. Truly therefore has it been said, that the salubrity of London in the nineteenth century and of London in the seventeenth is far greater than the difference between London in an ordinary season and London in the cholera.

But still we have had Cholera. In less than a quarter of a century we have had three visitations of this dreadful disease, which exhibits the essential characters of a pestilence of the middle ages; and if Typhus-gravior has disappeared, Typhus and its kindred diseases have taken its place; and the Registrar-General constantly presents before our eyes a faithful record of their ravages.

This is too true. We still have epidemics—and why? Because in all our towns there are large portions of the people who live in a state essentially the same as that which existed in the middle ages. The conditions are similar; the results are similar.

It is this unhappy class of people that form the exception to the general progress of the nation to which I have adverted.

These wretched places and their inhabitants do not obtrude themselves on the public eye. They are not seen in our common thoroughfares, nor in our splendid streets and squares. They are not known. The medical man knows them, the minister of religion knows them, the relieving officer knows them, a few dispensers of voluntary charity know them. They are not known to any one else.

Let me then describe one.

It is a small room, say twelve feet square; an inner room; no chimney, no window that will open, no inlet for fresh air, no outlet for foul air. There, on a miserable bed, lies a woman ill of typhus fever; a child at her side on the same bed is dying of that fever; a child already dead of it is stretched out on a table at the bed-side.

I could not breathe the air of that room. I could not remain in it long enough to write a prescription for the poor patients. As I was writing it at the street-door I shivered and felt sick. I knew that I had taken fever. I passed through a very severe form of it. I could take you to hundreds of such houses in every part of London; to hundreds of courts and lanes wholly consisting of such houses.

In such houses, with the conditions of the 15th and 16th centuries, Cholera, in the middle of the 19th, found and exerted a power similar to that which characterized the epidemics of the middle ages, and here Typhus and its kindred diseases continually hold their undisputed reign: houses whose unhealthfulness is increased by the only marks of the age which attach to them, their brick construction and their glass windows; those bricks and windows more effectually than the ancient wattles excluding the external, and confining the internal air, and thereby fostering the generation and spread of typhus. It is remarked by Dr Macculloch, in his account of the Hebrides, that while the inhabitants had no shelter but huts of the most simple construction which afforded free ingress and egress to the air, they were not subject to fevers, but when such habitations were provided as seemed more comfortable and commodious, but which afforded recesses for stagnating air and impurities, then febrile infection was generated. Houses in this state, without ventilation, without the means of cleanliness, worse than the huts of the savage, exist in great numbers in all our towns, and too truly merit the name they have acquired of "fever nests."

I once took a distinguished statistician of France to some of these places in London, and showed him the sick with typhus lying in their wretched beds; for the sick with typhus may be seen there every day of every year. After the painful inspection he exclaimed—"England is indeed adorned with a splendid mantle, but under it are concealed the greatest horrors."

Determined that this eminent person should see both sides of the picture, I next took him to the Model Dwellings.

What are the Model Dwellings? Small plots of civilization cultivated in the midst of a wide waste of barbarism.

In what does their civilization consist? In very simple matters.

The subsoil drainage of the site of the building;

The free admission of light and air to each inhabited room;

The abolition of the cess-pool, involving complete house drainage, an abundant supply of water, and the immediate removal by it of all refuse which it is capable of holding in suspension;

Means for the removal of house refuse not capable of suspension in water.

And this is all. And what are the results of these few and simple arrangements?

That the mortality among the inhabitants of these dwellings is less than that of London generally, and far less than that of some of the filthy and neglected localities in London, the Potteries of Kensington for example; while the mortality among children under ten years of age, on an average of three years, is one-half less than that of the nation generally, and four times less than that of the Potteries;

That there has not been a single death from typhus, or any other form of continued fever, among the adults in any of these buildings since their establishment; and that during the two first visitations of epidemic cholera, with the exception of two cases which occurred under peculiar circumstances, there was no attack of cholera in any of these buildings, while from four to six deaths from the pestilence occurred in single houses in the immediate neighbourhood.

Such are the results of the first imperfect attempt at improvement; which, remarkable as they are, are not more striking than the results of neglect. Of the children born in the best part of a town one fifth die before they attain the fifth year of age; of the children born in the worst, one-half die before they attain their fifth year. The inhabitants of the worst localities attain little more than one half of the age of those who live in the best. Of 100,000 children born in Surrey, 75,423 attain the age of ten years; 52,000 live to the age of fifty; and 28,878 live to seventy. In Liverpool, out of 100,000 persons born, only 48,211 live ten years; 25,878 live fifty years; and 8373 live seventy years. The probable duration of life in Surrey is 53 years; in Liverpool it is 26 years. Were the whole of the metropolis as healthy as the Model Dwellings, there would be an annual saving in London of nearly 20,000 lives. But these lives are not saved; this number of persons is allowed to perish every year, and they are as truly and as needlessly sacrificed as if they were taken out on Bethnal-green and shot.

When we bear in mind the suffering which in every case accompanies this waste of life, and the suffering which must inevitably follow it, and remember that it is admitted that these dreadful evils are remediable and preventible, it is difficult to suppress the natural feelings of indignation and of sorrow, that in a country calling itself Christian the application of the known remedies should be so long delayed.

It is right however to acknowledge that something has been done, and is in progress, for the improvement of the sanitary condition of the people. The principle is admitted that it is the duty of the Legislature to deal with this matter, and the first systematic legislative effort to bring about a better state of things has been made.

The Public Health Act is in operation, and the general and proper application by local authorities of the powers it confers would place every part of every town in Great Britain in as good a sanitary condition, at least, as that of the Model Dwellings.

Up to the present time (1855) there are under this Act 196 towns, containing a population of upwards of 2¼ millions. In about 50 of these towns, however, nothing has yet been done.

Eleven towns, with a population of about half a million, have adopted the powers of the Act in subsequent local acts.

Works of drainage and water supply are completed, or are in an advanced state, in 70 towns.

Mortgages have been sanctioned—

For drainage works and water supply,	nearly 1¾ millions sterling;
For private works of drainage and water supply,	about £45,000;
For paving, street improvements, &c.,	about £200,000;

Making a total of nearly two millions sterling devoted to sanitary improvement.[24]

24. This has been since greatly increased: see Appendix, p. 129. [ED.]

It is difficult at present to give the average cost of these combined and complete sanitary works; but the total expense for public and private works of drainage and water supply for houses of from £10 to £20 per annual rental, may be taken at 4d. per week per house.

The great obstacle to sanitary progress is the fear of rates, not so much on the part of the poor, who gladly pay for the improvements, but on the part of the owners of small tenements, by whom chiefly opposition is raised to the application of this Act.

In the town of Alnwick, public and private works of sewerage and drainage have been completed. There have been laid down about twenty miles of sewers and drains, and seventeen miles of apparatus for water supply, at a total cost, for the combined works, of 4d. per week per house for the term of thirty years; after the expiration of which period the cost of the works, both principal and interest, will have become liquidated, and the only expense thereafter will be for maintenance.

On inspecting these works, I saw in the tenements occupied by the lowest classes a high degree of cleanliness, wholesomeness, and comfort, and heard from the inhabitants an expression of the greatest satisfaction.

We have as yet no certain knowledge of the extent to which such works are capable of preventing sickness and lengthening life. But the most perfect drainage, combined with the most ample supply of water, will not alone secure for the public health all which it is practicable to accomplish. There must also be provision for the better construction of the houses of the poor; for the prevention of overcrowding; for street ventilation and cleansing, and for the exclusion from the neighbourhood of human dwellings of filth-creating animals and of noxious trades. When all this is done, as it might be done, and as it would be done were there a general perception of the crying evils it would remedy, Epidemics would disappear, the more formidable of them immediately, and all of them, I believe, in the end.

From the whole of these facts and observations we see—

1. That Epidemics are under our own control; we may promote their spread; we may prevent it. We may secure ourselves from them. We have done so. We have banished the most formidable. Those that remain are not so difficult to be conquered as those that have been vanquished. The causes

of Typhus are more completely under our control than those of Intermittent. We have banished Intermittent. We may put an end to Typhus. We have actually done so. We have encompassed the Model Dwellings by a barrier which neither typhus, nor even cholera, nor any of the other causes of excessive sickness and premature mortality have been able to pass. To the residents within that barrier the chance of life has been almost doubled; to their children it has been doubled; and compared with some other children of their own class it has been increased fourfold.

2. We see that Epidemics are not made by a Divine law the necessary condition of man's existence upon earth. The boon of life is not marred with this penalty. The great laws of nature, which are God's ordinances in their regular course and appointed operation, do form and give off around us, products which are injurious to us; but He has given us senses to perceive them, and reason to devise the means of avoiding them, and epidemics arise and spread because we will not regard the one, nor use the other.

3. We see that there are circumstances which render it doubtful whether civilization has yet attained a point that places it beyond the danger of retrogression. States in some respects of higher civilization than our own have relapsed into barbarism. There is indeed one circumstance which may give us hope; there is one humanizing principle which is now at least recognized and in partial operation, of which there is no trace in any nation of antiquity. I mean the principle of kindness as a governing influence, distinguished from the principle of brute force.

That the whole human race is one family, that the people of every colour, clime, language, government, and faith, are one brotherhood, and that the same law of love which is the bond of the union, strength, and happiness of a single family, is equally binding on the universal family of mankind, are the fundamental and distinguishing principles of our religion; and in proportion to our conformity in our private and public life to the spirit of these divine principles, advancement in civilization is certain; relapse into barbarism is impossible. But as yet there is no such conformity. We neglect the education of the people, quarrelling about the mode, and postponing the thing. We devote to a life of absorbing labour the child and the youth ungrounded in the elements of knowledge, untrained to habits of self-restraint, thereby dooming the man to the blankness and turbulence of ignorance and intemperance. We equally neglect the sanitary condition of the people. We make no provision for securing to the humblest classes, and they can make none for themselves, the conditions that are essential to their physical health, the loss of which to them involves and includes every other. We thus neglect body and mind, and then the disorders and vices which necessarily follow we endeavour to repress by punishments that harden but never reform, neither trusting nor trying the influence of gentleness, which our religion teaches us is stronger than ignorance, stronger than crime, and can master both. It is this state of things that places in danger the ark of civilization.

Lastly, we see the first step that must be taken to elevate the people: nay, even to bring them within the pale of the civilization already attained. We must improve their sanitary condition. Until this is done, no civilizing influence can touch them. The schoolmaster will labour in vain; the minister of religion will labour in vain; neither can make any progress in the fulfilment of their mission in a den of filth. Moral purity is incompatible with bodily impurity. Moral degradation is indissolubly united with physical squalor. The depression and discomfort of the hovel produce and foster obtuseness of mind, hardness of heart, selfish and sensual indulgence, violence, and crime. It is the Home that makes the man; it is the home that educates the family. It is the distinction and the curse of Barbarism that it is without a home: it is the distinction and the blessing of Civilization that it prepares a home in which Christianity may abide, and guide, and govern.

[The foregoing is from the Edinburgh Lectures. See Introduction. ED.]

QUARANTINE AND CONTAGION

[From First and Second Reports on Quarantine. See Introduction. ED.]

The object of quarantine is to prevent the introduction of epidemic diseases from one country into another, and its regulations are based on the assumption of the contagiousness of the diseases with which it deals; it being supposed that such diseases are propagated by contact, direct or indirect, of the unaffected with the affected. In accordance with this view the preventive means adopted by quarantine consist of the isolation of the sick or suspected, with whom it interdicts all communication, whether by person or by articles deemed capable of transmitting contagion.

When quarantine was first established, the spread of epidemic diseases exclusively or chiefly by contagion was a doctrine universally received;[25] but during the last century a change has gradually taken place in professional opinion in almost every country in Europe, particularly in France, Russia, and Austria, as well as in America, with respect at least to several of these diseases, chiefly by medical officers, who, having had the charge of the health of fleets and armies in different quarters of the globe, have been under the necessity of studying the circumstances connected with the outbreak and spread of formidable epidemics; and also by those who, having had the care of hospitals and dispensaries in large cities, have been obliged to visit the localities and abodes of the poorer classes, where these diseases are always the most prevalent.

<u>25</u>. The wide difference between the qualifications of the accomplished popular physician and the scientific investigator into the causes of epidemic sickness was strikingly exhibited in the first outbreak of Asiatic cholera in 1831, when the emergency required not merely a knowledge of the practice of medicine, but the power also of applying the philosophy of public health to the exigencies of the moment. How were these exigencies provided for?

A board, comprising all the most eminent and skilful physicians of the day, was assembled in the College of Physicians, under the presidency of Sir Henry Halford; and, after declaring, in opposition to the unanimous opinion of the physicians of Bengal, "that no measures of external precaution for preventing the introduction of the cholera morbus by a rigorous quarantine have hitherto been found effectual," they issued the following official notification:—

"To carry into effect the separation of the sick from the healthy, it would be very expedient that one or more houses should be kept in view in each town or its neighbourhood, as places to which every case of the disease, as soon as detected, might be removed, provided the family of the afflicted person consent to such removal; and, in case of refusal, a conspicuous mark, 'SICK,' should be placed in front of the house, to warn persons that it is in quarantine; and even when persons with the disease shall have been removed, and the house shall have been purified, the word 'CAUTION' should be substituted, as denoting suspicion of the disease; and the inhabitants of such house should not be at liberty to move out or communicate with other persons until, by the authority of the local board, the mark shall have been removed.

"It is recommended that those who may fall victims to this most formidable disease should be buried in a detached ground, in the vicinity of the house that may have been selected for the reception of cholera patients. By this regulation, it is intended to confine, as much as possible, every source of infection to one spot: on the same principle, all persons who may be employed in the removal of the sick from their own houses, as well as all who may attend upon cholera patients in the capacity of nurses, *should live apart* from the rest of the community.

"Whenever objections arise to the removal of the sick from the healthy, or other causes exist to render such a step not advisable, *the same* PROSPECT OF SUCCESS IN EXTINGUISHING THE SEEDS OF THE PESTILENCE cannot be expected. Much, however, may be done, even in these difficult circumstances, by following the *same principles of prudence,* and by avoiding all unnecessary communication with the public out of doors: all articles of food or other necessaries required by the family *should be placed in front of the house, and received by one of the inhabitants of the house after the person delivering them shall have retired.* Until the time during which the contagion of cholera lies dormant in the human frame has been more minutely ascertained, it will be *necessary,* for the sake *of perfect security,* that convalescents from the disease, and *those who have had any communication with them,* should be kept under observation for a period of *not less than twenty days.*

"All intercourse with any infected town and the neighbouring country must be prevented, by the best means within the power of the magistrates, who will have to make regulations for the supply of provisions.

"Other measures of a more coercive nature may be rendered expedient for the common safety, if unfortunately so fatal a disease should ever show itself in this country, in the terrific way in which it has appeared in various parts of Europe; and it may become *necessary to draw troops or a strong body of police around infected places, so as utterly to exclude the inhabitants from all intercourse with the country*: and we feel sure that what is demanded for the common safety of the state, will always be acquiesced in with a willing submission to the necessity which imposes it."

This announcement by the English physicians of 1831 was published throughout the land in the form of an Order of the King in Council. But the strong good sense of the public averted many of the mischiefs which these scientific advisers would have produced, had their counsels been carried into execution. The preventive measures which were eventually adopted by them consisted in prohibiting intercourse between one town and another by sea, and permitting it by land; thus, communication between London and Edinburgh by stage coach was perfectly free and uninterrupted, while communication between those capitals by sea was prohibited with such rigour that no interest, however powerful, could procure an exemption. Francis Jeffrey—at this time holding the high office of Lord Advocate of Scotland, and whose influence, from his personal and official connections, was very great—was unable to obtain permission for his faithful servant, in the last stage of dropsy, to go from London to Leith by water, lest he should carry with him to his native country, by that mode of conveyance, not the dropsy, which he had—but the cholera, which he had not.

"You will be sorry," writes Jeffrey to Miss Cockburn, "to hear that poor old Fergus is so ill that I fear he will die very soon. I have made great efforts to get him shipped off to Scotland, where he most wishes to go; *but the quarantine regulations are so absurdly severe, that, in spite of all my influence with the Privy Council*, I have not been able to get a passage for him, *and he is quite unable to travel by land*; he has decided water in the chest, and swelling in all his limbs. The doctors say he may die any day, and that it is scarcely possible he can recover."—*Cockburn's Life of Jeffrey*, p. 247.

These examples are not adduced for the purpose of casting obloquy on Sir Henry Halford, Dr Maton, and the other eminent physicians their colleagues, who vainly attempted to reduce to practice in the nineteenth century, the standard but obsolete doctrines taught, almost universally, in the medical schools in the country; but solely for the purpose of displaying the state of the science of Public Health in the year 1831–2, as far as the physicians of highest reputation and largest practice may be taken as its exponents.—*Origin and Progress of Sanitary Reform, by T. Jones Howell.*

The consideration of the common properties of pestilence, under whatever form or name it may occur, has led to the general conclusion that the true safeguards against pestilential diseases are not quarantine regulations, but sanitary measures—that is to say, measures which tend to prevent or remove certain conditions, without which pestilential diseases appear to be incapable of existing.

The whole machinery of quarantine is based on the assumption that by an absolute interdiction of communication with the sick, either by the person or by infected articles, it can prevent the introduction of epidemic disease into an unaffected community.

But this assumption overlooks the essential condition on which epidemic disease depends, namely,—the presence of an epidemic atmosphere, without which it is now generally admitted that no contagion, whether imported or native, can cause a disease to spread epidemically. Allowing, therefore, to contagion all the influence which any one supposes it to possess, and to quarantine all the control over it which it claims, there remains the condition, the primary and essential condition, which confessedly it cannot reach, namely, the epidemic atmosphere.

Experience affords evidence that the influence of an epidemic atmosphere may exist over thousands of square miles, and yet affect only particular localities. The cases of cholera which have occurred in numerous and widely distant parts of England and Scotland mark the presence of the epidemic influence; yet over this extended area cholera has fixed itself and prevailed as an epidemic only in very few places. Why has it localized itself in these particular places? Probably because it has there found conditions of a specific kind, either local or personal, or both. It follows that our true course is to make diligent search for all localizing circumstances, and to remove them, so as to render the locality untenantable for the epidemic. But quarantine makes no such search, and leaves all localizing conditions untouched and unthought of.

Hence the signal failure of quarantine as a means of prevention, with reference at least to the most prevalent epidemics, in all the nations of Europe in which it has been tried in modern times; and hence the general relaxation, and in some instances the total abandonment, of the system of quarantine, with reference to several diseases against which it was formerly rigidly enforced, and the growing distrust in the supposition that measures of this kind really afford protection against the introduction of any epidemic disease into any country.

The influence of great epidemics is not limited to human beings; it extends to all classes of domestic animals.

It is stated by Dr Thomas Lesslie Gregson, who was at Alexandria during the prevalence of the great plague of 1836, on duty there as surgeon-in-chief to the Naval, Military, and Civil Hospital, that cattle were attacked with decided symptoms of plague some time before the disease broke out among the human species. "Before the disease broke out," he says, "a number of the Pacha's oxen were seized with a malady, of which above one hundred died in a few days. I was sent to investigate and report on this epidemic. On examination I found gastroenterite in the most intense degree; so much so, that I have found extensive gangrene in oxen that have only been observed ill twelve hours. They had also large buboes. This I reported plague, and caused them to be interred deeply."

Quarantine is based on the assumption that epidemic diseases depend upon a specific contagion; but the question of contagion has no necessary connection with that of quarantine. The real question is whether quarantine can prevent the extension of epidemic diseases, whatever may be their nature, whether contagious or not. If it can, it is valuable beyond price; if it cannot, it is a barbarous encumbrance, interrupting commerce, obstructing international intercourse, periling life, and wasting, and worse than wasting, large sums of the public money.

But if the power of protecting the country from the introduction and spread of disease, whether contagious or otherwise, claimed by quarantine, be really possessed by it, this must be proved by other considerations than those which establish the contagiousness of disease; it is a mere matter of evidence and experience, and consequently the disputed point of contagion should be placed entirely out of view in this discussion, and the whole question should be argued on the broad ground whether or not quarantine is a public security, or is capable of affording practically any useful result.

There is indeed one point of view in which it may be proper, and even necessary, to consider the question of contagion with relation to that of quarantine. Assuming the existence of contagion, if it can be proved that quarantine, instead of affording any protection against contagion, absolutely fosters it, then the stronger the proof of contagion the more decisive the argument presented by it against quarantine; and it will be shown hereafter that this is the true and the only relation in which contagion stands to this question.

There is no more reason why the controversy on contagion should complicate the question of quarantine than why it should continue to encumber the general subject of the removable causes of disease, from which efforts have long been made to disentangle it.

The discussion whether epidemic diseases arise and spread from contagion or from common or specific poisons generated in the localities in which these pestilences first break out, has nothing whatever to do with quarantine, the sole inquiry with reference to this question being whether, however epidemic diseases arise, quarantine can prevent their introduction into a country or arrest their progress when there.

Few will question that the progress of the opinion of observers in Europe during the last half-century has been steadily towards a material modification, if not an entire abandonment, of the doctrine of contagion with reference to the majority of epidemic diseases, taking the word contagion in its strict sense, that is, the communicability of disease exclusively by contact: direct, that is, with the body or breath of an infected person; or indirect, with something which an infected person has touched.

Cholera may be taken as an example of the diseases of the epidemic class. When cholera first invaded Europe in 1831,[26] the belief in its contagious nature was almost universal, and in this country in particular there was scarcely a medical man who did not entertain this conviction; but as in India, where this disease is known, the belief in its contagious nature is universally abandoned, so in Europe it gradually diminished in proportion as opportunities of observing the disease increased; and now in Russia, Poland, Prussia, France, Belgium, and England, the contrary view, with few exceptions, is maintained.

26. See note p. 61.

There has been much confusion of terms in respect to the use of the words contagion and non-contagion. Professional men have avowed their belief of the contagiousness of typhus, and stated that they had experienced it in their own persons. When asked for the evidence on which the belief was founded, they have usually related some circumstances showing, not the contagiousness, but the infectiousness of the disease. Contagion is a term applicable to a different set of circumstances. According to the hypothesis of contagion, no matter how pure the air, no matter what the condition of the fever ward, if the physician only feels the pulse of the patient, or touches him with the sleeve of his coat, though he may not catch the disease himself, he may communicate it by a shake of the hand to the next friend he meets; or that friend, without catching it himself, may give it to another; or if the physician wash and fumigate his hand, but neglect the cuff of his coat, he may still convey the deadly poison to every patient whose pulse he feels during the day. If this were so, the track of a general practitioner who attended one patient labouring under a specific epidemic disease would be marked by the seizure of the rest of his patients; if it were true of cholera and typhus, the members of the General Board of Health must have fallen by these diseases, who from morning until night received inspectors that came from places where these epidemics were rife; and if any disease of common occurrence really possessed such powers of communication and diffusion, it is difficult to conceive how it is that the human race has not been long since extinguished.[27] To assume the method of propagation by touch, whether by the person or of infected articles, and to overlook that by the corruption of the air, is at once to increase the real danger, from exposure to noxious effluvia, and to divert attention from the true means of remedy and prevention. It is not in human power to take from any disease the property of contagion, if this property really belongs to it; but it is in our power to guard against and prevent the effects of any contagion, however intense; and it is equally in our power to avoid communicating to common disease an infectious character, and aggravating it into pestilence.

27. In January, 1866, the members of the Aberdeenshire Cattle Plague Association being much interested in the question as to how the disease could possibly have reached Pitmillan, Fovernan, no suspicious communication by beast or otherwise having taken place with the farm for weeks, Mr Hay, veterinary surgeon, inspector for the county, gave the following explanation of the matter in a letter to Mr Barclay, the hon. secretary:—"I am happy to be able to satisfy the public mind as to how the disease was brought to Pitmillan. About Christmas Mr Fraser got from Mr Duncan, flesher, Aberdeen, a quantity of beef rolled up in packsheet, which had apparently paid several visits to London round carcases, and doubtless mingled there with many of its kind from various places of the kingdom. After being removed from the beef at Pitmillan, this packsheet was thrown aside for some time, when one of the servant girls took and used it (unwashed) as an apron for a considerable period before the first cow got bad, and was carrying the kail in it to the cow after she was taken ill. You see by this that we are liable to get the disease at any time. Tons of packsheet return

weekly by railway, and no surer agent could be employed to bring rinderpest to the country." The secretary having some doubt about the guilt of the packsheet (which however, was gravely accused in both Houses of Parliament), reported his opinion that the contagion was conveyed by the wind! [ED.]

If indeed the emanations thrown off from the living body formed permanent and powerful poisons, like miasms connected with the products of decomposition, and if they were, like such products, capable of being conveyed unchanged to great distances, we should be able to live only in solitude; we could never meet in society, for we should poison each other; the first symptom of illness would be the signal for the abandonment of the sick, and we should be compelled by a due regard to self-preservation to withhold from persons afflicted with disease every kind and degree of assistance that required personal attendance.

Happily, we are not so constituted, and the evidence that has been adduced of the narrowness of the sphere even of the most virulent contagion, shows the groundlessness of the alarm sometimes entertained respecting this dreaded agent, while it points to the certain means of destroying it. The London Fever Hospital is separated from the Small-Pox Hospital only by the space of between thirty and forty feet, and the windows of the wards of both establishments are immediately opposite each other: yet there is no instance of the communication of small-pox to the typhus patients, nor of typhus to the small-pox patients; nor of either disease to the convalescent, or to the official inmates of the adjoining establishment. There does not appear to be a single instance on record, in any country, of the extension of infection beyond the walls of an hospital, or even of a lazar-house, so as to injure in any manner the nearest inhabitants.

But though it appears that modern experience and research have shed considerable light on the origin and progress of epidemic diseases, yet there are still some circumstances connected with their propagation which the present state of our knowledge does not enable us to understand, and which therefore appear to us as difficulties.

These cases are sometimes termed exceptional; but they are only apparent, not real, exceptions; as in all other departments of human research, they are merely indications of the imperfection of our knowledge, and advancing science will unquestionably one day so elucidate these very exceptions, as to render them additional confirmations of the true conditions.

In the present state of popular opinion it has been deemed requisite to enter into this detailed consideration of the general subject of contagion, because it appears that in proportion as undue weight is attached to this dreaded agent the effect is mischievous; since, "it diverts attention from the true source of danger, and the real means of protection, and fixes it on those which are imaginary; creates panic; leads to the neglect and abandonment of the sick; occasions great expense for what is worse than useless; and withdraws attention from that brief but important interval between the commencement and the development of disease, during which remedial measures are most effective in its cure."

It is also necessary to examine the questions of contagion and quarantine apart from each other, because there are points of obscurity, and therefore grounds for controversy, which, in the present state of our knowledge, may be reasonably considered as belonging to the former, that do not attach to the latter. The inquiry with reference to quarantine, indeed, is simple, and lies in a narrow compass. The sole question to be determined is, whether or not it accomplishes, or is capable of accomplishing, its professed object, and this is a mere question of evidence and experience.

The object of quarantine is to prevent the introduction of epidemic diseases from one country into another, and the agency which it employs for this purpose is the isolation of the sick; the detention of, and the placing under inspection for a given period, persons who come from an infected country or district, though they may not be actually sick; and the purification of articles of commerce presumed to be capable of imbibing and conveying pestilential virus, before such articles are landed and dispersed.

It appears that facts and observations place beyond all reasonable doubt the utter inutility of this system.

If there be any truth in the preceding representation, that epidemic diseases are universally and inseparably connected with an epidemic atmosphere, the question is at once decided. Quarantine can exercise no more control over this epidemic atmosphere than over the electricity and temperature of the common atmosphere, and the direction and force of the wind.

If it be true that epidemic diseases, such, for example, as influenza and cholera, traverse the globe in determinate courses or zones, and often spread from country to country, and through the vast populations of their great cities, in single weeks, and even days, it must be futile to array such a machinery as that of quarantine, that is to say, a vessel placed at the entrance of one or two seaport towns, a line of soldiers guarding a few miles of the frontier, of a particular country against morbific agents, which pursue their course like the blight that destroys the vegetation of a country in a night, and which extend their influence over the greater part of the habitable globe.

If it be true that the epidemic influence precedes the actual outbreak of epidemic disease—that that epidemic influence is present in a country, creating a predisposition or susceptibility to disease before the epidemic appears in its true and recognized form,—quarantine must be futile, because, before it takes its precautions or erects its barriers, such as they are, the epidemic is already in the country busy in action, vitiating the blood of the most susceptible of the population, and preparing the way for its general attack.

If it be true, as ancient and modern authorities are agreed, that, without the essential preliminary of an epidemic atmosphere on the spot, foreign contagion is inert, and that, unless both concur, no pestilence ensues, quarantine under any circumstances must be useless; for in the absence of an epidemic atmosphere it must be useless, because then no disease will spread beyond the individual affected; and with the presence of an epidemic atmosphere it must be useless, because then the disease will spread wherever the infected atmosphere goes and finds favouring conditions.

If the preceding principle be true, it must be futile to place vessels coming from infected countries in quarantine, unless those vessels are capable of bringing with them an epidemic atmosphere, and unless quarantine can control such an atmosphere when imported; and the uselessness of this procedure will be placed in a still stronger light when recent experience as to the comparative insusceptibility of Europeans, though resident on the spot, to plague itself is considered.[28]

28. Dr W. H. Burrell, Deputy Inspector-general of Hospitals, who was three years Principal Medical Officer at Malta, presented, in 1852, to the General Board of Health, an elaborate examination on the plague which had formerly raged in that island. The following are the conclusions to which he had arrived:—

"1. There is no evidence to prove, or even to render it probable, that the plague was introduced either into Malta in 1813 or into Gozo in 1814 by importation.

"2. There is every reason to believe that the plague existed in Malta at the time of the arrival of the ship supposed to have introduced the disease; and that in Gozo the first case (a stranger) contracted the disease from local causes, which enhanced by quarantine, produced it in others.

"3. The lower orders, and those occupying the lowest, most crowded, and worst ventilated dwellings, furnished the great majority of cases; which decreased in proportion with improvement in these respects.

"4. As this discriminative preference of the disease to attack certain classes, living in certain localities, never obtains to the same extent with diseases arising from a specific contagion, it is more than probable that the causes engaged in the generation of the plague are not constant, but variable and accidental; its initial cause, the peculiar atmospheric constitution, having no power to develop the disease, unassisted by season and local conditions.

"5. The transmissibility of plague from person to person out of the noxious atmosphere in which it originated—the only certain test of such a power—has not been proved by the four instances, during thirty-eight years, in which it is alleged to have been communicated to persons employed by the Quarantine Department of Malta, carbuncular affections being endemic among the population of this island.

"6. Quarantine restrictions enforced by the penalties of *corporal punishment* and *death*, and seconded by the greatest dread of contact with suspected persons or things, among the panic-struck populations of Malta and Gozo, utterly failed to arrest the progress of plague; on the contrary, where these restrictions were carried to their utmost limits by an absolute power, there the disease persisted longest, and the mortality was greatest."

"All these circumstances," says the French Dr Chervin, speaking of the restrictions and cruelties of quarantine, "are calculated to fill with horror the breast of every feeling and honest man; and we are really obliged to offer violence to ourselves in not giving vent to our indignation against the partisans of contagion, who yet desire to continue to defend their erroneous opinions, and who, to this day, have used all their efforts to make obscure and disfigure the subject, to the great detriment of truth;—who have never ceased to deceive governments, which think it their duty, with regard to this disease [Yellow Fever], to surrender themselves to the judgment and knowledge of medical men,—who have never ceased to describe it as contagious, and have induced those authorities to adopt, with respect to it, the most false and contrary measures, and to neglect the suitable, prophylactic, and *preservative* means, and others which might have put an end to the disastrous epidemics of this disease;—thus it is they have always acted contrary to truth, to the interest of governments and of humanity."

"I am of opinion," says Dr Reece, of New York, "that the oppressive features of our quarantine system should be reckoned among the relics of barbarism which an enlightened Legislature should make haste to abrogate for the sake of our character as a people. There is no pretext for the perpetuation of a system founded in ignorance, and fruitful only in public and private injustice, cruelty, and wrong."

"Cholera," says Professor Caldwell, of America, "though a fatal scourge to the world, will, through the wise beneficent dispensation under which we live, be productive of consequences favourable alike to science and humanity. Besides being instrumental in throwing much light on the practice of physic, it will prove highly influential in extinguishing the belief in pestilential contagion, and bringing into disrepute the quarantine establishments that have hitherto existed."

If the great practical truth, taught by modern investigation and experience, be, that the only real security against any kind and degree of epidemic disease is an abundant and constant supply of pure air, the prevention of overcrowding, and the dispersion of the sick; and if, as is generally agreed, confinement in a foul atmosphere can convert common fever into pestilence, and ventilation and dispersion can dissipate any contagion, then quarantine must be not only useless but pernicious, since the invariable effect of quarantine as hitherto practised in all countries has been the congregation and confinement of the sick, and of those who, though not actually sick, are suspected to have in them the seeds of disease, requiring only a few days or hours for their development,—the congregation and confinement of such persons in a limited space, often in a filthy ship and an unhealthy locality, and always under circumstances calculated to excite apprehension and alarm—conditions in the highest degree favourable to the generation and spread of disease: it follows that quarantine, instead of guarding against and preventing disease, fosters and concentrates it, and places it under conditions the most favourable that can be devised for its general extension; and therefore must not only fail to accomplish its object, but tend to produce the very calamity which it endeavours to prevent.

***

The principal ground on which objection is made to the continuance of quarantine is that the fundamental principle on which it is based is fallacious, and that the only means of preventing the origin and spread of epidemic disease is the adoption of sanitary measures. Substitution of sanitary measures for quarantine restrictions would render the importation of any disease from one country into another in the highest degree improbable.

There has been and continues to be a popular impression of the importation or the contagiousness of disease, created by the frequent occurrence of epidemic diseases amongst itinerant classes of the population. Seeing the occurrence of such diseases amongst those who travel, it is an easy and apparently a natural inference that the diseases are carried by them. Thus, the low tramps' lodging-houses in our towns were in the Sanitary Report shown to be throughout the country the worst of fever-nests in each place; but they were also shown at the same time to be the places where there was the most overcrowding and the greatest filth. With a stationary population, with the same overcrowding and filth, it may be confidently pronounced that the disease would be worse. When by bad weather the tramps are detained and kept stationary, it is worse. The tramping about from town to town and in the open air—the movement which to superficial observation imports the disease—in reality mitigates it. From what we have already said, it is consistent with this general statement that tramps infected with fever in one place may carry it with them and spread infection in another place amongst classes of persons predisposed by the like habits and conditions, as was exemplified in the spreading of the Pali plague. Of late times the poor Irish emigrants are said to have imported fever into this country; they are represented, for example, to have imported fever into Liverpool; but the description of the places where the fever burst out, and the overcrowding in them, displayed fever-nests sufficient to have produced fatal results on the most robust of the stationary populations. "In one small cellar with no window," a gentleman, who ministered to the wants of the poor people who had crept for shelter into damp uninhabited houses, and who, it was stated, fell a victim to the contagious nature of the fever, found "eighteen persons in fever, lying on wet dirty straw. In one house he counted eighty-one, in another sixty-one, in every stage of fever, on straw in the corners." It would be surprising if the poor Irish had not imported fever into the lower districts of towns, when, as in Glasgow, they have added 10,000 annually to the already overcrowded and wretched population of that city; just as the miserable refugees from the infected villages of Ragpootana carried the pestilence into the close, filthy, and already overcrowded huts of the neighbouring villages. But the conditions in which the Irish emigrants have arrived, and have been crowded together in the towns as well as on shipboard, are just the conditions in which fevers arise amidst stationary populations; and, we may confidently state, would have been worse had the particular class of migrants been stationary.

The like delusion as to the *importation* of disease is created by the appearance of fever amongst the migrants at sea. It is important that the universal effects of overcrowding, filth, and atmospheric impurity should be known and discriminated in all cases. It will be seen that they produce their effects at sea as well as elsewhere. It appears to be most important also to display the facts as to the common existence of the conditions of fever in ships themselves as at present regulated; and that, if properly regulated, instead of being fever-nests or "the means of importation" of the disease, a voyage in the open sea would become a sure means of arresting any such disease. Epidemic disease is often more severe in ships when stationary in port than when sailing, and with them the passage in fair weather when overcrowding is avoided is a means of mitigation.

The sanitary regulation of the ships themselves—a measure of the utmost importance to the seafaring classes of the community—would accomplish far more than could be hoped for or pretended to be accomplished by any known system of quarantine, and would have, moreover, a beneficial effect upon popular opinion by removing the fallacious appearances which favour the belief in imported disease, while they divert attention from the true causes of disease, the removable and preventible causes that exist on the spot.

The basis of sanitary legislation is the evidence that has been accumulated in relation to the whole of the epidemic, endemic, and contagious diseases, and the latest opinions of medical authorities with reference to them. It having been shown by indubitable evidence that the prevalence and mortality of typhus, scarlatina, cholera, and every other epidemic disease, are uniformly in proportion to the low sanitary condition of the population, the Legislature has decided on attempting to check the prevalence of these diseases by laying the foundation of sanitary improvement.[29] It appears that the measures adopted by the Legislature with this view should be consistently carried out and applied to the dwellings of all classes of the population whether on land or at sea. In the larger vessels in which well-directed care has been exercised, the general ill-health has been reduced below the average ill-health of populations of the like ages on shore; but from the evidence which has been brought from witnesses at the ports, medical men well acquainted from long practice in the mercantile marine, it appears that the *general* condition of merchant-vessels, and of the forecastle in which common seamen are, for the most part, lodged, renders them in effect cellar-dwellings, just as dark, foul, and unventilated, as the filthy, unaired, and dismal cellars on shore with which the Legislature has endeavoured to deal. It appears also that typhus and other epidemic diseases do break out at sea in these movable cellars, just as they do in the cellars of the dirtiest courts on shore; and were it not that seamen work in a purer external atmosphere, that they are below decks comparatively for short intervals only, and that in general they are men at the most robust periods of life, it is probable that epidemic disease would be still more frequent among them; an inference supported by the fact that whenever passengers, emigrants, and others are, owing to stormy weather, much confined to the berths below, some form of malignant disease is almost sure to break out.

29. See pp. 57, 129, works executed after this was written. [ED.]

There are not wanting instances in which the energetic adoption of such measures as were available, particularly the enforcement of all practicable means of cleansing, and the resolute removal of nuisances, warded off Cholera to a very great extent, even under circumstances in which a formidable attack appeared inevitable; and perhaps it may serve for encouragement and guidance to direct attention to one or two of such examples.[30]

30. The two following examples are taken from "Results of Sanitary Improvement," by Dr Southwood Smith, 1854. [ED.]

One of the most remarkable of these occurred at Baltimore, during the prevalence of epidemic cholera in America, in 1849.

The population of that city was about 149,000 souls. The site of the town is naturally salubrious, and parts of it are well built; but the districts near the river occupied by the poorer classes are low and damp, and liable to remittent and intermittent fevers, and, therefore, predisposed to cholera.

In the spring of 1849, the pestilence, which had attacked with great violence several neighbouring towns, appeared to be close upon the city. A general conviction prevailed, both among the authorities and the citizens, that uncleanliness had much to do with the development and spread of the disease; they therefore spared neither money nor labour to purify the city, and they gave the execution of the cleansing operations to experienced and energetic officers, who performed the work so vigorously, that it was generally admitted that never before had the town been in so clean a state, or so thoroughly purified, as during the summer months of the year 1849.

About the middle of June, while cholera was prevailing at New York, Cincinnati, and other places, north and west of Baltimore, diarrhœa broke out, and became general over the whole city, accompanied by another symptom which was universal, affecting even those who had no positive attack of diarrhœa; namely, an indefinable sense of oppression over the whole region of the abdomen, seldom amounting to pain, but constantly calling attention to that part of the body.

"At that time," says the medical officer of the city, "I felt assured that the poison which produced cholera pervaded the city; that it was brooding over us; that we were already under its influence, and I anticipated momentarily an outbreak of the epidemic. In about two weeks, however, from the commencement of this diarrhœa, and the prevalence of the uneasy sensation which accompanied it, these symptoms began to subside, and in a short time they wholly disappeared. Simultaneously with their disappearance, cholera broke out at Richmond, and other towns south of Baltimore. I then felt assured that the fuel necessary to co-operate with this poison did not exist in our city: that the cloud had passed over us and left us unharmed."

No case of cholera was reported to the Board of Health or other authorities of the town as having occurred during this time; but on close examination, it was ascertained that four deaths had taken place from the disease in its most virulent form.

That the cholera poison had really pervaded the city, was appallingly evinced by an event which occurred in its immediate vicinity.

The Baltimore almshouse is situated about two miles from the city, on sloping ground, remarkable for its beauty and salubrity, in immediate contiguity with the country-seats of several of the wealthy families of the town. It is surrounded by a farm of upwards of 200 acres, belonging to the establishment, for the most part under cultivation. The building is capable of accommodating between 600 and 700 inmates. An enclosure of about five acres, surrounded by a wall, adjoins the main building upon its north side. In the rear of this north wall is a ravine, which at one point approaches the wall to within about nine feet. This ravine is the outlet for all the filth of the establishment. It is dry in summer, but retentive of wet after rain. The space between the wall and the bed of the ravine is not under tillage, but is overgrown with a rank, weedy vegetation, common in rich waste soils. The physician of the establishment, under the same apprehension of an outbreak of cholera as had prevailed in Baltimore, had taken the same precautions against the disease, and had placed the establishment itself in a state of scrupulous cleanliness.

On the first of July cholera attacked one of the inmates. On the seventh a second attack occurred. This was followed in rapid succession by other seizures, and within the space of one month 99 inmates of the establishment had perished by cholera.

Within the building and grounds the most diligent search failed to discover anything that could account for this outbreak; but on examining the premises outside the northern wall, there was found a vast mass of filth, consisting of the overflowings of cesspools, the drainage from pigsties, and the general refuse of the establishment. "In short," says the medical officer, "the whole space included between the ravine and the wall, upon its north side, was one putrid and pestilential mass, capable of generating, under the ardent rays of a Midsummer sun, the most poisonous and deadly exhalations."

During the greater part of the time that this outbreak continued, a slight breeze set in pretty steadily from the north, conveying the poisonous exhalations from behind the north wall directly over the house.

The first persons attacked were those who happened to be particularly exposed to the air blowing from the north side of the building.

On the male side of the house there was no protection from the ravine. The female side was partially protected by three rows of trees. The residents on the women's side were more numerous than on the men's, but the attacks were considerably less.

Among the paupers, those who slept in apartments exposed to the north were attacked, those not so exposed generally escaped.

In the basement story of a building, opening directly to the north, and close to a spot which received the contents of one of the cesspools, 17 lunatics were lodged, all of whom were attacked, and all died.

Eight medical students were attached to the establishment, of whom four occupied apartments with a northern exposure, and four were lodged in rooms with a southern exposure. The four whose rooms were exposed to the north were attacked, the four whose rooms were not thus exposed escaped.

The manager, also, who slept in a room above that of the students looking to the north, was attacked: his family, whose rooms looked to the south, escaped.

Men, after some difficulty and delay, were employed to remove the filth and drain the ravine, the whole surface of which, after having been thoroughly cleansed by a stream of water, was thickly covered with lime, over which was put a deep stratum of earth. The men employed in this work were attacked with cholera, as were some of the several inmates of the almshouse who had been dispersed throughout Baltimore, but the disease did not spread to any other persons in the city. From the 25th of July, the day on which the drainage was completed, the disease suddenly declined from 11 the day previous, to 3, and, by the 9th of August, had entirely disappeared.

***

In the case of Baltimore, and the Baltimore almshouse, a neglected spot was severely visited by the pestilence, while, by well-directed exertion, an entire city escaped. In our own country an instance has lately occurred (1854) in which, by similar exertion, a particular spot escaped, while a populous town was devastated by the plague.

No town in Great Britain has ever been so severely visited by cholera as Newcastle, yet the garrison of Newcastle has wholly escaped.

The barracks in which the garrison of Newcastle is quartered are situated about three-quarters of a mile from the centre of the town. In houses at distances varying from 20 to 200 yards of the barrack gates, numerous deaths from cholera took place, and in a village 250 yards from the barracks the pestilence prevailed to a frightful extent for many days, numbering one or more victims in almost every cottage.

On the outbreak of the pestilence in the town, the medical officers of the garrison, with the sanction and assistance of their superior officers, exerted themselves with great promptitude and energy to carry into effect all the means at their command, calculated to lessen the severity of an attack from which they could not hope altogether to escape. The sewers, drains, privies, and ashpits were thoroughly cleansed; all accumulations of filth were removed; the spots where such filth had been collected were purified; the freest possible ventilation was established day and night in living and sleeping rooms; overcrowding was guarded against; the diet of the residents was, as far as practicable, regulated; the men were strictly confined to barracks after evening roll-call, and were forbidden to go into the low and infected parts of the town; amusements were encouraged in the vicinity of the barracks; every endeavour was made to procure a cheerful compliance with the requirements insisted on, without exciting fear; and there was a medical inspection of the men twice, and of the women and children, once daily.

The influence of the epidemic poison upon the troops was demonstrated by the fact that among 519 persons, the total strength of the garrison, there were 451 cases of premonitory diarrhœa, of which 421 were among the 391 men, irrespective of the officers, women, and children, the attacks being in some instances obstinate, and recurring more than once. Yet such was the success of the judicious measures which had been adopted, that no case of cholera occurred within the barracks during the whole period of the epidemic; and every case of diarrhœa was stopped from passing on to the developed stage of the disease: while in Newcastle there were upwards of 4000 attacks, and 1543 deaths.[31]

<u>31</u>. Results of Sanitary Improvement by Dr Southwood Smith, 1854.

The case of the "Eclair," and the history of the Epidemic Fever which occurred at Boa Vista in 1845, have been declared by high medical authority to afford "conclusive evidence that Yellow Fever is sometimes imported." It will therefore be necessary to make a careful examination of the circumstances relative to this Epidemic.

It has been affirmed, and generally credited, that unusual effort has been made to ascertain the facts of this case under circumstances more than commonly favourable to the discovery of the truth. Two official Reports respecting it, drawn up after personal inspection on the spot, have indeed been presented to Parliament—one by Dr McWilliam, and the other by Dr King; and several official notices of these reports have been published; but the evidence on which these two Reports were founded was not collected until some time after the cessation of the epidemic. The statements of witnesses, for the most part poor and ignorant, many of whom had a direct interest in establishing the importation of the disease by a British ship, have been admitted implicitly, even with respect to dates and circumstances not of recent occurrence, and without due examination of the credibility of their testimony; and on all material points the reporters have arrived at directly opposite conclusions.

On a review and comparison of the whole of the statements which have been made with respect to this case, it appears that the steam-ship "Eclair," with a crew of 140 officers and men, proceeded in 1844 to the coast of Africa, and was stationed for upwards of four months (130 days) at the island of Sherboro, with a view to blockade the eastern outlet of the passage at Shebar. This place is considered one of the most unhealthy on the African coast; vessels remaining near the island very rarely escaping an outbreak of Yellow Fever on board. The land is represented as low lying, some parts being marshy, and the rest thickly wooded, and abounding in rank vegetation.

According to the account of the surgeon of the "Eclair," Mr Maconchy, the ship on this occasion was anchored at the mouth of the river, in position where she "was surrounded with filthy-looking river water, urged backwards and forwards by the tides through extensive tracts of mangrove bushes." The fresh water used on board was also bad, holding in solution a quantity of offensive vegetable matter, which produced in some of the crew attacks like mild cholera. The men, in parties of from 30 to 40, were often sent up the river on boating expeditions, where they remained for seven or eight days at a time exposed, "whether they slept on board or ashore, perhaps after a hard day's labour, to all the exciting causes of fever, and a tainted nocturnal atmosphere, in the rainy season, heavy weather having set in, and the men constantly getting as wet as possible."

The danger of this boating service is thus stated by Dr King:—

"The duty in boats up African rivers involves considerable risk at any time of the year, but it can never be practised in the rainy season without endangering the health and lives of all who are employed, and such were evidently the sad consequences of the boat expeditions of the 'Eclair.'"

The crew, according to Mr Maconchy, in addition to this dangerous service, and the dreariness and monotony of the situation, were exposed to another depressing agency, "from seeing the prizes of other ships passing frequently to Sierra Leone, whilst they considered themselves out of the reach of such good fortune."

Another cause was probably in operation even at this time, namely, the foul condition of the ship, as will hereafter appear.

Under these circumstances, fever broke out on board the ship, and proved fatal to ten of the crew; eight of the ten deaths being considered by the medical officers as directly consequent on the boating expeditions. Though there were other and severe cases of sickness on board, these deaths appear to include the whole of the ship's mortality during her stay at Sherboro, a period, as has been stated, of above four months.

In the month of July the "Eclair" left this station, returned to Sierra Leone, and anchored in the harbour, where she appears to have remained 13 days. This happened to be the rainy season. The crew went on shore, where several of them remained at night unable to reach the ship from being in a state of helpless intoxication.

The consequences were soon apparent. While the ship remained in the harbour, fever again broke out on board with great violence, and continued without intermission during this and the following month. In this sickly state she again left Sierra Leone, proceeded northward in company with another ship, the "Albert," and anchored in the Gambia on the 10th of August "(one of the most unhealthy months at that place)," where she remained until the 15th. All this time, the fever steadily increasing, she arrived on the 21st of August at Boa Vista. She had now lost, since leaving Sherboro, 13 more of her crew, making in all, from the first outbreak of the disease at Sherboro, 37 attacks and 23 deaths; that is, 1 in 6 of the crew had died.

On anchoring in the harbour of Boa Vista, pratique was at once offered to her commander, Captain Estcourt, but he replied that he could not think of accepting it until he had communicated the state of his vessel to the authorities on shore. After some deliberation the Governor-General consented to the landing of the ship's company, in the hope that the formidable disease, by which so many had already perished, and so many others were still placed in imminent danger, might be checked. Accordingly the crew, both the healthy and the sick, were sent to a Fort on an islet a mile distant from the town (Porto Sal Rey), and the officers were lodged in the town itself. This took place on the 31st of August.

The hope of benefiting the crew by the change of their quarters from the ship to the land was not realized. On the contrary, the sickness continued to increase with so much virulence that, at the end of the third week after the arrival of the ship at Boa Vista, no fewer than 60 fresh cases were added to the sick list, and some deaths took place nearly every day.

In this state of things a consultation of the medical officers was held on the condition of the crew, the result of which was a recommendation that the ship should immediately proceed to Madeira, and if the fever received no check, that she should go on to England. In conformity with this advice, the whole of the crew, the sick as well as the healthy, were forthwith re-embarked, and the ship sailed from Boa Vista on the following day, namely, the 13th of September.

The sequel to this sad narrative shows that no improvement took place during the passage of the "Eclair" to Madeira, where she was refused pratique. She therefore proceeded next day on her voyage to England, and anchored off the Isle of Wight, at the Motherbank, on the 28th of

September, having lost, since sailing from Boa Vista, 12 more of her crew. Thus in the short space of 37 days, that is, from the time when she anchored at Boa Vista on the 21st of August, till her arrival at the Motherbank on the 28th of September, there occurred no less than 90 attacks and 45 deaths, including the death of her excellent and devoted captain.

On her arrival in England the ship was put in quarantine, and remained under the direction of the Privy Council until the 31st of October.

On the day following her arrival, Dr Richardson proposed that the sick should be immediately removed to a wing of Haslar Hospital, to be appropriated exclusively for them; stating, that in his opinion, if the sick were placed in well-ventilated wards, with fresh bedding, and the other means of cleanliness afforded by an hospital, there would be no further risk to the attendants than would occur in wards set apart for cases of typhus fever.

To this advice, Sir William Pym objected, and instead of allowing the removal of the sick, he ordered the vessel, with the whole of her crew, to proceed from the Motherbank to the Foul Bill Quarantine Station at Standgate Creek, which place she did not reach until the afternoon of the 2nd of October, that is, four days after her arrival at the Motherbank, where they remained six days more before their removal into another vessel. Thus were all on board detained close prisoners in a pestilential atmosphere on the shores of their native land; their anticipations that at length they should quit the scene of such terrible sufferings, and of so many horrors, their hopes of life and health, totally destroyed. The consequence was, that within these ten days, five more deaths took place, nor was it until the Lords of the Admiralty declared their conviction that the only means of preserving the lives of the survivors of the crew would be the entire removal of every individual from this ill-fated ship, that they were permitted to quit it. Their removal took place on the 8th of October, after which event two more deaths occurred, one of them being that of the pilot who took the vessel from the Motherbank to Standgate Creek.[32]

> 32. A striking contrast to this treatment of the crew of the "Eclair" is exhibited in the case of Her Majesty's frigate, the "Arethusa," which recently (Feb. 14, 1852) arrived at Plymouth from Lisbon, having on board cases of small-pox. Instead of putting the ship in quarantine, and confining the healthy in the same poisonous atmosphere with the sick, wiser counsels on this occasion prevailed, and more humane measures were adopted. On the advice of Dr Rae, Inspector of the Royal Naval Hospital, the sick, twelve in number,

were immediately removed to that establishment, and of these two died, without any communication of the disease.

As already stated, official inquiries were directed to be made into the causes of this extraordinary mortality, from which it appears:—

That there was nothing peculiar in the disease itself. The medical and other officers of the ship, as well as the medical and other officers at Boa Vista, that is, all competent witnesses who actually saw the disease, concur in stating that it was nothing more than an aggravated form of the common endemic fever of the African coast; a view which is decisively confirmed by the original description of the disease in the medical journal of the ship, and by post-mortem examination.

In opposition to this generally-received opinion, however, Sir William Pym promulgated a statement that, in addition to the common African fever, the celebrated *nova pestis* of Dr Chisholm had been introduced into the vessel by a passenger taken on board at Sierra Leone; this disease being, as he represents, a fever *sui generis*, known by the name of the African, Bulam, Yellow, or Black Vomit Fever, attacking the human frame but once, and differing from the common remittent fever in being highly contagious.

That the doctrine on which Sir William Pym's assertion rests met with little countenance from medical authorities is apparent from the statement of Sir William Burnett, who says:—

"The whole of this, as regards the peculiar properties of the disease, called by Sir William Pym, Bulam, &c., is a gratuitous assumption on his part, and, in my opinion, has no foundation in fact; and in my view of this part of the subject I am supported by nineteen-twentieths of the medical officers of both services, who are of opinion with myself that the more ardent form of Yellow Fever is a mere modification of the bilious remittent so extensively known all over the tropical regions."

He adds: "The fever which prevailed in the 'Eclair' was unquestionably a remittent fever, originating in marsh miasmata, and the exposure of the men in boats during rainy weather."

Dr King and Dr Stewart, in official Reports upon this case, state their concurrence with Sir William Burnett. Dr McWilliam, on the other hand, is of opinion that the disease, though primarily an endemic remittent of the African coast, became, from a series of causes, exalted into a concentrated remittent or Yellow Fever, and in that manner acquired new and peculiar properties, not primarily and essentially belonging to it.

With reference to this latter opinion, it may be observed that the Governor-General of the Cape de Verd Islands affirms, that not one of those who with a view to escape the pestilence emigrated to the different islands of the Archipelago, had the disease, or communicated it to others. According to the view of Dr McWilliam, therefore, this disease must have been of a very singular character, for in its origin at Shebar, it was not contagious, at Boa Vista it became contagious, while in the other islands of the Archipelago, wherever the sick or the uninfected fled, it again laid aside its contagious character, and did not spread to a single individual.

All the inquirers and reporters agree in stating that among the causes which concurred in communicating to this disease so extraordinary a degree of prevalence and mortality, the more important were the following:—

The employment of the crew uninterruptedly for an unusual length of time, including the sickly season, in a peculiarly unhealthy situation, and dangerous local duty.

The exposure of men, whose systems were impregnated with the seeds of disease imbibed in this unhealthy locality, to the risks of unrestricted liberty on shore, in the atmosphere of Sierra Leone, during the rainy season; one consequence of which freedom being their "inordinate indulgence in ardent spirits of the worst description."

And subsequently, at Boa Vista, the confinement of the crew, the sick as well as the uninfected, in a place still more crowded, filthy, and unventilated than their quarters on board, instead of their dispersion in a pure atmosphere.

Some conception may be formed of the unfavourable circumstances under which the crew were placed at the Fort, from the account which, on personal inspection, Dr King gives of its sanitary condition, who states that from the absence of all means of cleansing, from the actual accumulation of filth, and from the impossibility under any circumstances of obtaining a free circulation of pure air, owing to the plan of the building, the atmosphere which the sick, the convalescent, and the healthy were compelled to breathe, day and night, must have been polluted and deleterious in the extreme; and that into a space incapable of affording sufficient accommodation for 50 men, upwards of 100, including the sick, were huddled together under a most oppressive heat, the thermometer ranging from 81° to 86°. This description is confirmed by the testimony of Dr Almeida, who states that having been requested by the Governor-General to go to the Fort and see the sick, "he found them so extremely crowded that he could hardly pass between them."

The influence of such conditions in conducing to the virulence and spread of the disease has been already exemplified in what has been stated under the head "Localizing Causes;" but it must be added, that the crew had here also access to ardent spirits, in which both the sick and the uninfected indulged to still greater excess even than at Sierra Leone.

"It is with great regret," says Sir William Burnett, "I have now to state on the best information, that while in this situation means were found to supply the sick as well as others with enormous quantities of ardent spirits, which were drunk with avidity and produced the most deleterious effects; indeed, I have reason to believe that some were absolutely killed by it as if by poison. Had there not been a fever already in existence, the intense heat (86° of Fahrenheit), the nature of the soil, and this dreadful intoxication together, would have been fully sufficient to have produced it, and one of the worst kind too, in which irritability of the stomach and dark-coloured vomiting would have been conspicuous symptoms."

The actual result, as stated by Dr McWilliam, was that the accession to the sick-list and the mortality became much greater at this time than they had been at any previous period, and that from an endemic remittent of the African coast, the disease became exalted into a concentrated remittent or Yellow Fever.

Indubitable evidence further shows that, in addition to all these causes of disease, the crew when on board were constantly inhaling a poison generated in the ship itself. On a superficial examination the ship may have appeared clean, and Sir William Pym positively asserts that she was so; but there is conclusive evidence that this appearance was fallacious.

From the records of the Medical Department of the Navy have been extracted the following decisive statement with reference to this point, by Captain Simpson, late of the "Rolla:"—

"In June, 1845, being then in command of the 'Rolla,' I went on board the 'Eclair' off Shebar River. Commander Estcourt reported to me that he had sent a boat up the Sherborough River, and that the crew, during night, were exposed to heavy rain and much lightning, and were sick: some deaths had occurred on board. In the early part of July I went to Sierra Leone for supplies; the 'Eclair' was there; the vessel was anchored close to the shore; and I advised her Commander to move her further out, which he did. There seemed much excitement amongst the crew; some liberty had been given them, and drunkenness and sickness were the consequence. Wood was received on board for fuel in lieu of coals. This wood was green, as I understood at Sierra Leone, and very unhealthy to burn."

This fact is substantiated by the log of the "Eclair," which shows that from July 16th to the 19th inclusive, the crew were employed at Sierra Leone in wooding.

The influence of a quantity of greenwood recently taken on board a ship navigating the tropical seas, in producing destructive fever, is shown in the most striking manner by the history of the "Regalia," and by that of the "Vestal."[33]

33. For these cases see the Second Report on Quarantine, pp. 64, 299.

Further evidence will be found in the Medical Department of the Navy to show "that the hold of the 'Eclair' was in a pestiferous state;" and Dr King states, that long after the people left the ship in England, and when the engines were removed, mud, some inches deep, was found under the flooring.

"I should scarcely have noticed the above circumstance," he says, "but for some remarkable occurrences which took place in the same vessel at a subsequent period, which confirmed me in the opinion I had previously formed that the origin and continuance of the fever on board depended solely on local causes.

"The 'Rosamond,' formerly the 'Eclair,' was commissioned at Woolwich on the 5th of November, 1846, for the Cape of Good Hope station, but none of the former crew rejoined the ship. During the time of fitting out, four cases of typhus fever occurred, and were sent to the hospital, where two of them died, but it is necessary to mention that typhus was prevalent at Woolwich at the time. The steamer left England for the Cape on the 23rd of February, 1847. Three days after sailing, one of the men was affected with slight febrile symptoms, and he continued more or less indisposed for a number of days, but occasionally felt so well that he returned to his work. After the ship entered the tropics, however, the disease began to assume a new and alarming character; and when off the Island of St Nicholas, and almost in sight of Boa Vista, the man died, having had for two days previous black vomit and other characteristic symptoms of Yellow Fever. Within a few days afterwards the 'Rosamond' arrived at Ascension, where I was then stationed; and Commander Foot having communicated to Captain Hutton, the superintendent of the island, every particular respecting the illness and death of the seaman, I was ordered, with Dr Sloane, the surgeon of the hospital, to make a report on the case, and at the same time to suggest measures for the benefit of the ship without endangering the health of the people on the island. Having obtained from Dr Slight, surgeon of the 'Rosamond,' every information relative to his late patient, we stated our opinion that the disease the man died from was sporadic Yellow Fever. * * * On the following morning I went on board with the view of learning something to enable me to form an opinion as to the sanitary condition of the ship, and for the purpose also of inspecting the sick, as the surgeon informed me he had then a suspicious case, with symptoms of a low kind of fever. I had barely time to take a cursory view of the after parts of the ship, when my attention was called to the patients, who were all mustered in the steerage, and I found the man the doctor had alluded to in such a precarious state that I recommended him to be sent on shore immediately. The only other severe case was that of a supernumary lad, who was taken ill the same morning, but the indications of a low malignant fever were so apparent even at that early stage, as to induce me to express my opinion to the surgeon that he would not probably survive 24 hours. As it was most desirable to prevent a panic among the ship's company, I went on shore to consult with Captain Hutton, and make arrangements for their reception. * * * The patients themselves attributed their illness to foul air in the forepart of the ship; one of them said he suffered so much from an abominable stench in the boatswain's storeroom, that he represented the circumstance and obtained permission to cut a hole in the floor, which exposed to view a considerable quantity of soft mud, and five or six buckets full of it mixed with decayed shavings, and emitting an offensive odour, were removed at the time.

"It appears then, that besides an unusual number sleeping in the fore-cockpit, some of them at least had been exposed to a morbific miasma, exhaled from a festering mass of filth in the bottom of that part of the ship. The quantity of mud, no doubt, was small in comparison with what had accumulated when the vessel arrived at Spithead from the coast of Africa, yet the malaria eliminated from that small and circumscribed focus was equally virulent in its operation, and produced the same disease in a few who were placed within the sphere of its influence."

Such is a brief narrative of the circumstances connected with this ship and her crew.

But it has been alleged that while the landing of the crew of the "Eclair," at Boa Vista, afforded no benefit to the ship's company, it inflicted a grievous evil on the inhabitants of the island; that several individuals in contact, or close proximity with the sick, became affected with the same kind of fever; that from these individuals the malady spread to others with whom they came in contact, and from these again to others, as from so many centres of contagion, until the disease became general over the island, thus affording a positive instance of the importation of epidemic disease. The alleged facts on which these representations rest are the following:—

It is stated, that during the occupancy of the Fort by the crew, there was a small Portuguese guard stationed there; that this guard was several times relieved; that at the time when the "Eclair" left the island, the guard consisted of one negro and two European soldiers; that within three days after the sailing of the "Eclair" both Europeans were attacked with fever similar to that from which the crew of the "Eclair" had suffered; that the negro soldier, who, with his comrade—the man sent from Boa Vista to nurse the two Europeans—on returning from the small island to Porto Sal Rey, had been—"as a matter of precaution"—"restricted for ['about 8' or] 17 days to the occupation of a small hut at the northern end" of the town, was afterwards attacked,—though not confined to bed until the day following his return to barracks; and that a woman (Anna Gallinha), who lived next door to this hut, was the first person who was attacked with fever in the town. It is further stated that a man (Pathi), who had been a labourer on board the "Eclair," was also attacked with fever, according to one account, on the day after the "Eclair" sailed; but according to another account, on the third day after that event.

Such are the alleged facts, and the only ones bearing directly on the communication of a specific contagion by the crew of the "Eclair," collected by Dr M'William by personal inquiries on the spot; and these, in his opinion, present a chain of evidence sufficient to establish a positive instance of the importation of epidemic disease.

With reference, however, to these inquiries, it has been already stated that they were not instituted until several months after the departure of the "Eclair" from Boa Vista;—the only regular practitioner on the island (Dr Kenny) who could have given authentic and trustworthy information respecting the nature and progress of the disease, had died;—the witnesses examined by Dr M'William, poor and ignorant, gave their evidence, hearsay and otherwise, in the loosest possible manner;—their statements as to dates and occurrences, alleged to have happened several months before the inquiry took place, were received implicitly, without examination into the correctness of their answers and the credibility of their testimony;—all the witnesses of this class appear to have spoken under the influence of the strongest feeling of self-interest, with a view to establish a claim to pecuniary compensation should they be able to make out a case against the "Eclair," in which expectation they were not disappointed, since the sum of £1000 was eventually granted by Great Britain for the benefit of the inhabitants;—and to this motive may probably be ascribed the highly coloured and exaggerated statements put forth by these people on the re-appearance of fever in the following year.

Taking the facts, however, precisely as they are represented in the Report of Dr M'William, they do not, as the proof of the allegation in question requires, present a clear and palpable chain of evidence, connecting as cause and effect the fever of the ship with the epidemic on shore; but, on the contrary, there is not a single link undoubtedly connecting the one with the other.

Take the first case forming what is represented as the first link in this presumed chain, the seizure with fever of the two guards at the Fort. Two European soldiers lately arrived in the colony, and therefore peculiarly predisposed to an attack of endemic fever, go from Boa Vista, which at that time was healthy, to a confined, unventilated, overcrowded, and filthy spot on another island, where fever was raging to such a degree that within the space of three weeks there had occurred no less than 60 attacks and 33 deaths, in a crew consisting on the arrival of the ship of 117 officers and men. There is in this no evidence of the propagation of disease by a specific contagion; on the contrary, it is the ordinary production of disease by its ordinary cause, namely, exposure to a polluted atmosphere, the pollution being, in this instance, excessive from overcrowding; from accumulation of filth; from foul and offensive privies; from the impossibility of the admission of fresh air, owing to the construction of the building, and from the intense and oppressive heat, the thermometer ranging from 81° to 86° of Fahrenheit. The seizure of two men with fever under such circumstances is precisely analogous to the attack of persons, previously healthy, with typhus, who take up their abode in the crowded and filthy courts and alleys of English towns.

Take the next link in the chain, the attack of the negro soldier. The circumstances respecting this man, being precisely the same as those relating to the two other guards, the same answer would have sufficed for both, but according to the testimony of the man himself, his illness was very slight, and his companion who was sent to lodge with him at the hut in Porto Sal Rey, had no illness at all during the whole time of their seclusion.

The third link in the chain is the presumed fact, that a woman (Anna Gallinha), who lived next door to the hut in which these two men had been confined, was seized with fever soon after they had left it, and that she was the first person attacked, at least whose illness attracted public attention, in the town of Porto Sal Rey. Dr King states, that on a personal examination of the soldier who had experienced the slight attack of fever, he said that during the seventeen days that he and his companion were confined to the hut, "they had no communication with any one." Dr M'William, on the other hand, affirms that Gallinha was a frequent visitor at the hut, and, indeed, cooked for the men. Supposing Dr M'William's account to be the correct one, it is surely more reasonable to attribute the attack of Gallinha to the local causes to which she was exposed, and which Dr M'William admits were sufficient to account for her illness, than to contagion derived from a man whose illness was so slight that it had not confined him to his bed for a single day, and which was incapable of infecting his companion who was constantly with him night and day.

"By the time Anna Gallinha was taken ill," says Dr M'William, "much rain had fallen; the weather had become more hot, and, in short, there now (but not before this) existed the recognized elements for malarious evolution."

"In that part of the town called Beira, or Pao de Varella," reports Dr King, "where Anna Gallinha and the soldiers resided, the houses are of the lowest description, and the people who occupy them are generally very poor and destitute; there is a large pool of stagnant salt and fresh water immediately behind; but to windward of this part of the town, and still nearer to the houses, there is a locality which is resorted to by many of the people when obeying the calls of nature; and the exhalations from the one, and the effluvia from the other, are blown by the north winds in the direction of Beira."

A similar description of this locality is given by Dr M'William,—

"In the upper portion of the town," he says, "which is called Pao de Varella, the houses are in general mere hovels, rudely built, and much crowded together, and with few exceptions dirty. They are occupied by the lowest classes. From the total absence of any police laws the streets here are also very filthy."

Here then were present in full force, as is admitted, the ordinary localizing causes of fever; to which it is more consistent to refer this case, than to an extraordinary and foreign cause.

But at this point the presumed chain of evidence stops; the chain is suddenly snapped; there is no further link traceable; there is nothing really connecting the illness of Gallinha with the next cases, or with the general spread of the disease which rapidly followed, and we need hardly state, that in order to prove the spread of a pestilence by contagion, communication, either direct or indirect, must be proved to have existed between all the persons attacked.[34]

<u>34</u>. The widow of the next victim (Affonso) denied his having had communication with Gallinha; and Dr Almeida "found about 20 people sick" in Porto Sal Rey only three or four days after Gallinha's death. It is evidently more rational to ascribe these numerous attacks to epidemic influence, which it is admitted was now present, than to contact with this woman, for the fact of which there is in truth not a shadow of evidence.

For the only other case of fever that is stated to have occurred shortly after the sailing of the "Eclair," namely, that of the labourer (Pathi) who had been employed on board the ship, will scarcely be considered as affording an additional link; since admitting that this man contracted his fever while employed on board the "Eclair," his case would be merely one of infection from going on board a foul ship, a generally recognized cause of fever:—

"Whenever," says Dr Stewart, "fever has prevailed much in ships on the West India and African stations, strangers going on board of those ships have been particularly liable to its attack; but on sending fever cases from those ships to the hospitals and private houses on shore, it has not been found that the disease extended from them."

But as in the locality of the dwelling of Gallinha, so in the district in which this man lived, there were local causes abundantly sufficient to account for the endemic origin of his disease. He resided in Rabil, one of the hamlets in the neighbourhood of Moradinha, at some distance from Porto Sal Rey. Of this locality Dr King says:—

"If there is one spot more than another in the whole island where, from its physical peculiarities, endemic fever might be expected to begin first, and end last, that locality is Moradinha, and the villages in its vicinity, in one of which Pathi resided."

It may be observed further, that whatever may have been the cause of this man's fever, it is admitted, that for three weeks at least it was communicated to no one else in the house at Moradinha, where he was attacked, and remained for eight days, and not to any one else in that neighbourhood for 11 weeks; that his illness was extremely slight, and that on his return to his own house no disease broke out for some time in his family. According to Dr M'William, the first member of his family that was attacked was one of his children, who was taken ill "on the tenth or eleventh day" after his return, the illness of this child being gradually followed by that of two other children. But Dr King affirms that these children were not taken ill until "about a month" after their father's return, and that it was not until the succeeding month (the middle of November) that his wife was seized, "when the disease was general throughout the island." It is also particularly to be observed, that a child in another family at Rabil, having no communication with the family of Pathi, died about the same time as Pathi's first child, and that the disease broke out at least as early at Rabil as at Porto Sal Rey.

Lastly, it may be urged in opposition to the opinion that the contagion was communicated by the crew of the "Eclair," that the small island on which the sick were landed and to which they were confined was a mile distant from the town of Porto Sal Rey, and that on reference to the map attached to Dr M'William's report, it is obvious that the North-east trade wind must (according to the theory of Sir William Pym, as applied to the Neutral Ground at Gibraltar in 1828) have dispersed the contagion if in existence, or carried it in a contrary direction from Porto Sal Rey.

***

For a more minute examination of the cases of the guards at the Fort, and of Pathi and others, as presented by Dr M'William, we refer to the Note of Dr Browne, Appendix No. III. (p. 306),[35] who has there shown the real value of these cases, considered as links forming a chain of circumstantial evidence.

<u>35</u>. *Vide* the Report itself.

The authentic facts attending the intercourse of the ship's company with the inhabitants of the island, afford further evidence that no infection could have been communicated by the former to the latter. Thus, it is admitted that Captain Estcourt, the commander of the ship, went directly from the infected vessel to reside with Mr Macaulay, the judge: no infection was communicated to Mr Macaulay, or any part of his family.

The officers of the gun-room—midshipmen, warrant, and engineer—on disembarking from the ship, took a house for themselves and their servants in the town, and mixed unreservedly with the inhabitants: no infection was communicated to any individual with whom they had intercourse.

The crew obtained or took leave to pay frequent visits from the small island to the town of Porto Sal Rey, where, according to Dr M'William, they resorted chiefly to the house of one Georgio, who kept a spirit store; the only consequence of which visit, considered by Dr M'William a remarkable one, appears to have been that this man (and "shortly afterwards" two females who associated with them) was attacked with headache and general fever on the evening of the day he was visited by the

"Eclair's" people; a result which admits of a more obvious solution than the communication of febrile contagion on the part of persons who were themselves in perfect health.

The soiled linen of the officers and crew having been brought on shore on the first arrival of the vessel, was immediately given out to be washed to the washerwomen of Porto Sal Rey, and the careful search made after these women, brought to light no fewer than seventeen persons who were so employed.

"The soiled clothes," says Dr King, "linen, cotton, and flannel, which had accumulated in the officers' cabin from the time of their departure from Sierra Leone, were contained in at least 12 bags, which were taken on shore at Porto Sal Rey the same evening the ship arrived, and distributed next morning (22nd August) to the washerwomen of the town. Now, if the disease possesses the power of reproduction, its poison must [according to general opinion] have been as certainly communicated through the medium of *fomites* as by direct contact with the sick on board or at the fort; yet none of the washerwomen nor any in their families were attacked with fever until November, showing an interval of 70 days after exposure to the infection."

That it was not from any want of susceptibility to the influence of febrile poison that these women escaped the danger of this exposure to *fomites* was proved by subsequent events; for during the progress of the epidemic, all of these women, according to Dr McWilliam, with only one exception, were attacked with the prevailing fever; two between six and seven weeks after the sailing of the "Eclair;" five, two months; two, three months; three, four months; and one, five months afterwards.

"None of the deaths," says Dr M'William, "took place until fever was general in Porto Sal Rey, so that in none of these cases can the occurrence of the fever be fairly attributed to infectious matter conveyed by the linen."

The Guards at the Fort were many times relieved, and the soldiers were sent direct from the small island to their barracks in Porto Sal Rey, without conveying any disease to their comrades. On one occasion two soldiers who are stated to have lived in a room next to that in which the sick of the "Eclair" were lodged, on being taken ill, were conveyed at once to the barracks, yet they infected no one in their quarters.

From a list drawn up by Dr King, of the names of the islanders who were engaged as labourers on board the "Eclair," it appears that there were in all 63 persons employed in coaling, watering, and cleansing the ship. These men appear to have had unrestricted communication with the ship's crew. According to Dr M'William, the whole of these labourers went to their respective homes every night, except those from Estacia and the Eastern villages, who generally slept at Porto Sal Rey. None of these men were themselves attacked with fever, excepting one (Pathi) whose case has been already considered; none of them communicated fever either to their own families or to the persons with whom they lodged in the town, yet subsequent events proved that they as well as the washerwomen were sufficiently susceptible subjects, since, during the progress of the epidemic, the greater part of them were attacked by the disease; none, however, within a month after the departure of the "Eclair;" a few within two months, but the majority not until four or five months afterwards.

That the geographical position of the Cape de Verd Islands places them within the legitimate domain of Yellow Fever, and that this disease is no stranger to these islands, is admitted on all hands. According to Dr M'William,

"The north-western part of the island, where Porto Sal Rey is situated, is low and flat, and almost wholly occupied by sand, which, blown up from the north-western shore through the water-courses, and other hollows, accumulates in mounds twenty and thirty feet high, which are drawn about and shifted by any little variation of the direction of the wind."

On the flat between Porto Sal Rey and the village of Rabil, which is about four miles to the southward of Porto Sal Rey, Dr M'William states that there is a point where the sea, when the waves are high—

"Breaks over the elevated beach, and penetrates through the shingle, so as to accumulate, and run inland in the form of a narrow creek, from 200 to 300 yards from the sea-shore. During the rainy season, this, in common with the other flats on the island, is inundated to a considerable extent, as is evident from the appearance of the soil in those places not covered with sand, as well as by the presence of a rude raised causeway, which the people have constructed over part of the hollow flat, to render it passable during the rains. * * * Near the town is a hollow flat, spread over an area of about a mile, with the same soil and subsoil as that in the town. The central part of this area is occupied by a salt pan, which contains not less than 300 troughs, each a foot deep, and about thirty feet square, into which the salt water is poured, there to evaporate and form salt. During and for some weeks after the rainy season, the whole of this space is more or less inundated. * * * The water is left to stagnate on the Rabil side, and as it dries up during the hot weather, little alluvial islets are from time to time exposed, which the people avail themselves of to raise a small crop of corn. Indeed the greater part of the ravine, from Rabil downwards, is in a state of rude cultivation, and contains large green fœtid pools, with all kinds of decomposing matter, the effluvia from which was most offensive when I was there in May, 1846."

Experience has shown, that such a condition of sandy soil is as fruitful a source of endemic and malignant fever as a marsh or swamp. Dr Lind, who wrote nearly a century ago, expressly notices the unhealthiness of Boa Vista, particularly during the rainy season, stating that, "strangers who arrive here at this season are liable to be visited by a general sickness," and instances its white sand as a mark of an unhealthy locality. Dr Fergusson confirms the correctness of this indication of insalubrity.

"That sandy soils," he says, "should, in malarious climates, prove as productive of aggravated remittent fever as the swamp, has never been sufficiently explained. Certain it is, however, that they do so, in a marked and prominent degree. The Alemtejo and Algarve of Portugal—regions, I may say, altogether of sand—are the most prolific of fever of any in the Peninsula."

Another instance is found in the unhealthiness of Vera Cruz, which is spoken of by McCulloch in the following words:—

"It is said to be the original seat of the Yellow Fever." [Bulama?] "The city is well built and the streets clean, but it is surrounded by sand-hills and ponds of stagnant water, which, within the tropics, are quite enough to generate disease. The inhabitants and those accustomed to the climate are not subject to this formidable disease; but all strangers, even those from the Havannah and the West India Islands are liable to the infection. No precautions can prevent its attack, and many have died at Xalapa, on the road to Mexico, who merely passed through this pestilential spot."

Dr King states, that if ever endemic fever derives its origin from a vitiated and malarious state of the atmosphere, Boa Vista abounds with the elements for its production. Among these he enumerates swamps and pools of stagnant water, in the immediate vicinity of Porto Sal Rey, and over the whole district of Rabil; patches of rich alluvial soil near the other villages, the recognized sources of noxious exhalations; the wretched food of the lower classes, and still more, the polluted atmosphere which they breathe in their crowded and ill-ventilated abodes, and the general disregard of cleanliness in their houses and streets, "a combination of morbid causes," he says, "which would produce malignant fevers in any part of the world."

The relative position of Boa Vista to the African coast would further naturally lead to the expectation that it must be subject to diseases of the same character, and no one disputes that this is the case. The residents of the island, military, medical, and civil, concur in stating that endemic, bilious remittent fever, prevails there more or less every year; that there is no season in which it does not carry off several of the inhabitants, and that it often prevails epidemically.

"The testimony of the most intelligent men in the island," says Dr King, "including Dr Almeida, Senor Baptista (the Consul's agent), the Mayor of Rabil, the Judge of Fundas Figieras, and the Judge at Old Town, removes every doubt as to the fact that fever prevails to a certain extent, and carries off several of the inhabitants in the months of November and December every year; and this endemic fever, which recurs annually, and which Dr Almeida calls the bilious remittent, does not always present the same mild aspect and character; on the contrary, it is well known that in certain years the disease was epidemical, and in comparison with other seasons, very fatal."

Dr M'William records the fact, that such epidemic seasons occurred and proved unusually mortal in the years 1821–2, in 1827, and in 1833.

It is most material to a right understanding of this whole subject to observe, that a Yellow Fever Epidemic had broken out at this very time in an adjoining island, St Jago. It is stated by Dr Stewart, in his Report in the Admiralty Correspondence, that "in the adjoining island at Porto Praya, there was Yellow Fever whilst the ship was at Boa Vista." Captain Simpson states that it recurred in the following year at Porto Praya; "is common there at times and quite endemic."

That co-incident with the presence of the "Eclair" at Boa Vista one of these epidemic seasons was impending, was declared by the usual indications, which in warm climates precede and accompany such visitations. These premonitory signs on this occasion were a great fall of rain at an unaccustomed season; the consequent accumulation of large quantities of stagnant water in and about the towns and villages; the occurrence of extraordinary heat; the prevalence of light winds with frequent calms rendering the weather extremely sultry and oppressive; the appearance of sporadic cases of fever of more than common intensity; the almost simultaneous outbreak of pestilence amongst cattle and other domestic animals; and the visitation in greater numbers than common of destructive insects.[36]

36. See note, p. 16.

These prognostications were so manifest as to excite the attention and alarm of the intelligent classes of residents. The Governor-General states:—

"Great falls of rain took place at a very advanced period of the season, which remained stagnant."

The British Consul says:—

"Up to the month of October, extraordinary heat and the fall of a large quantity of rain had been experienced, events which were surprising to the oldest inhabitants."

The British Judge says:—

"Stagnant water had settled in great quantity at the back of the town, to which was joined great heat in the weather."

Dr King says:—

"The information received on the island in 1846, fully corroborated what is stated in the above extracts, the periodical rains, contrary to what usually happens, did not set in till late in September. In October, November, and December the winds were light and variable, with frequent calms, and the weather became in consequence extremely sultry and oppressive. The grass and green crops were nearly destroyed by the long previous drought, and what little appeared after the rains was devoured by the locusts, which visited the island in greater numbers this year than was ever known to be the case before."

Though Dr M'William, on his inspection of the island with a view to ascertain the true cause of the pestilence, took no notice of any of these premonitory signs of its approach, Sir William Burnett was fully aware of their signification, and calls special attention to one of the most important of them in his Report to the Lords of the Admiralty.

"I beg to lay before their Lordships," he says, "an extract of a letter from the Governor-General of the Cape de Verd Islands, and likewise extracts of letters from Mr Macaulay and the British Consul, residents on the island of Boa Vista, distinctly showing the very remarkable state of the weather preceding the attack of the inhabitants of the island, which very important circumstance in a case of this kind I regret to observe Dr M'William has omitted to take any particular notice of."

The event foreshadowed by these occurrences rapidly followed. As early as the middle of September a few cases of unusually malignant fever broke out, but, as has been already stated, the first case that attracted public attention occurred on the 12th of October; a few others followed during the remainder of this month; a still greater number broke out in the beginning of November, and the epidemic came to its height in the latter half of November, continuing to prevail throughout December, and recurring for several months in the following year.

As in epidemic outbreaks in general, so in this instance, individual or sporadic cases occurred some time before the appearance of the epidemic in its true and proper form. On minute inquiry, it was discovered that one if not two cases occurred as early as the 14th of September (Pathi), another on the 20th of September (Roque), and a third on the 21st of September (Agostinho): no other cases, at least none that attracted attention, appeared to have occurred until the one already mentioned (Gallinha), on the 12th of October. These sporadic cases all occurred in the ordinary localities of epidemic disease, and among individuals belonging to the classes that usually furnish its first and chief victims.

At Boa Vista, in addition to other proofs of the presence of a stagnant and pestilential atmosphere, there was the evidence derived from the prevalence of unusual sickness and mortality among domestic animals.

"That the common air," says Dr King, "which was inhaled by every living thing on the island was in an epidemic condition in the months of October, November, and December of both years, is sufficiently demonstrated by the simultaneous occurrence of universal sickness and great mortality among the cattle (including horses, cows, mules, donkeys, and goats) at the very time that fever was raging among the inhabitants. And, further, there was this remarkable coincidence, that after an interval of some months and the disappearance of the disease both in man and beast, the same fever broke out again in the towns and villages about the rainy season of the following year, and was again accompanied by the same murrain among the cattle, which in the two seasons proved fatal to two-thirds of the whole stock of the island."

These considerations afford all the evidence which the nature of the case admits of, that the sickness which affected the island on this occasion arose, not from the landing of the sick of the "Eclair," but from climatic and endemic causes.

To sum up the whole of this case, then, it appears that the evidence in favour of the allegation that fever was imported into Boa Vista by the "Eclair," amounts to this: that four men, not of the ship's crew, were attacked with fever while performing military service in a locality in which no fewer than 60 of the crew themselves were seized; that one man not of the ship's crew who worked as a labourer on board the ship "about eight" or "two" days, had a slight attack of fever, while 62 men also not of the ship's crew, and who also in like manner worked as labourers on board the ship a longer time, were wholly unaffected; and that a month after the sailing of the vessel, a woman was attacked with fever who happened to be a next-door neighbour to two of the soldiers who had served on duty at the Fort—one of whom was unaffected, and the other not even confined to bed—simultaneously with the children of the labourer (Pathi) who resided in one of the dirtiest localities of the island.

Against such evidence, if evidence it can be called, must be weighed the following countervailing considerations:—

It is admitted that the "Eclair" had been exposed on the coast of Africa to the causes which usually develope epidemic fever in that country; that intensity was given to those causes by circumstances which occurred at Sierra Leone, where she took in green wood as fuel, and where her men went on shore during the rainy and sickly season, and indulged in the unlimited use of ardent spirits; that her hold was in a pestiferous condition, and that a quantity of putrid mud had collected between her timbers. It is proved that the fever which broke out under these circumstances was the common endemic African coast fever, which, it is admitted, is not contagious, and which is assumed to have become contagious on this particular occasion, expressly to account for its alleged importation. It is admitted that on the landing of the ship's crew at Boa Vista, though the men mixed freely with the islanders,—though the officers lodged in the town,—and though, when some of them became sick, they were nursed by the inhabitants,—there was no communication of the disease in a single instance. It is admitted that of seventeen washerwomen who washed the linen of the officers and crew, not one became infected, although all these women, except two, suffered severely from the disease at subsequent periods after the epidemic became general. It is admitted that with the exception of one case, which has been proved on inquiry to have been no real exception, 87[37] labourers worked on board or in the neighbourhood of the ship daily, and returned to their homes at night, without taking any precautions,—without becoming themselves infected,—and without communicating infection to any individual of their families;—though, like the washerwomen, the greater part of these men suffered severely when the epidemic became general. It is admitted that the Cape de Verde Islands are within the Yellow Fever zone, and are liable to frequent and severe outbreaks of epidemic fever. It is admitted that the physical and social conditions of Boa Vista are eminently those which are found by universal experience to localize epidemic diseases whenever an epidemic influence is present. It is admitted that the "Eclair" arrived at Boa Vista at the season of the year when endemic fevers usually prevail. It is admitted that at the very time of her arrival, Yellow Fever was actually prevailing at Porto Praya, in the island of St Jago, into which it is not alleged that the disease had been introduced by importation. It is admitted that some time before the outbreak of the epidemic, the atmospheric and other conditions which usually precede and accompany the development of epidemic disease, were so manifest as to attract general attention. It is proved that sporadic cases of the disease appeared, as is usual, some time before the presence of the epidemic was declared in its distinct and recognized form. It is admitted that the epidemic influence extended to animals as well as man, a mortal epizootic disease prevailing over the whole of the island at the same time. It is proved that the epidemic did not break out until about a month or six weeks after the "Eclair," with all her crew, healthy and sick, had left the island. It is admitted that a similar epidemic appeared among men and animals the following year, not imported, but entirely of local origin.

<u>37</u>. The aggregate number of the lists furnished by Dr M'William.

A consideration of these circumstances has satisfied most of those who have inquired into the case, that the arrival of the "Eclair" at Boa Vista with fever among her crew, and the occurrence of a similar disease on the island, were mere coincident events, and that the appearances which might at first view have given some colour to the notion of importation were fallacious.

Among those who arrived at these conclusions were—The Governor-General, who says:—

"The disease was perfectly endemic. Not one of those who emigrated to the different islands of the Archipelago had the disease or communicated it to others. It did not make its appearance till a month after the departure of the steamer.... The disease had its origin in the great falls of rain which took place at a very advanced period of the season, and which remained stagnant in the neighbourhood of the place."

Mr Rendall, the Consul, who says:—

"The competent officers of the 'Eclair' at all times pleaded that the fever which had appeared and rested on board was nothing more than the 'common African coast fever;' the opinion of the medical men on the spot continued to be that the fever was merely the common African fever, and that no danger existed of its spreading among the people."

Mr Macaulay, the Judge, who says:—

"So long an interval had elapsed between the departure of the 'Eclair' and the appearance of the first serious case of fever in the town, that we were all disposed in the first instance to attribute it, as well as the general sickness of the place, rather to stagnant water, which had settled in great quantity at the back of the town, joined with the great heat of the weather and the dirty state of the streets. The 'Eclair' had left Boa Vista nearly a month before any case of fever exhibited itself in the town.... No injury whatever had resulted from the unrestricted intercourse which had subsisted during the whole of the 'Eclair's' stay in the harbour, between the officers and men (not in the hospital at the fort) and their friends on shore."

Captain Simpson, who says:—

"If I give my opinion on the fever that was on board the 'Eclair,' I should say it commenced at Shebar: and it was to be expected that men being exposed in boats to night duty during the rains, would be sickly; that it was likely to be much increased at Sierra Leone by the long continuance of the vessel there, and the men having leave to go on shore during this season, when this place is so very unhealthy, and seamen always so incautious; the occupation of the 'Eclair's' officers and ship's company on board the 'Albert' in clearing the holds, at all times a very dangerous work in the Tropics; and the use of green wood for fuel. In fact, I should have been very much surprised if the 'Eclair' had not been sickly."

Sir William Burnett, who, in reporting on the case to the Lords of the Admiralty, says:—

"After a careful perusal of the papers he (Dr M'William) has sent, I am compelled to say that I cannot conscientiously arrive at the conclusion the Doctor has done, namely, that the fever was occasioned by intercourse with the 'Eclair.'"

Sir William Burnett adds, with reference to the general question of importation:—

"With respect to the importation of the disease into various places, except in one instance, and that even is surrounded with doubts (I mean that of Her Majesty's sloop 'Bann'), I entirely disbelieve it. Both the surgeons of Bermuda Hospital most distinctly deny on two occasions that the epidemic which prevailed in 1843 was imported or contagious; I have also caused the medical reports of Jamaica Hospital for more than twenty years to be examined; and though hundreds of patients with yellow fever in all its most appalling forms, including black vomit, &c., have been treated in that establishment, not one of the medical officers in charge of the hospital have ever hinted at the disease being contagious; and if it be needful I can cite numerous other instances."

As to the apprehension that the crew of the "Eclair" might have imported the disease into England, he says:—

"I have no hesitation in declaring my firm belief that the sick men of the 'Eclair' when that ship arrived at the Motherbank, might have been landed at Haslar Hospital and placed in the well-ventilated wards of that establishment without the public health suffering in the smallest degree. It is a fact well known, and of the truth of which I can give the most satisfactory proof, that during the autumn of every year merchant-ships arrive in our harbours loaded with the produce of the coast of Africa, having perhaps lost great part, nay in some instances the whole, of their crew by the fever of the country; or some are still labouring under fever when the ship arrives in the Thames, and are sent to the hospital in that state; yet no instance is known of any infection having been produced by such procedure; in fact it is perfectly certain that it never did take place."

Dr King, who says:—

"The inhabitants in general are firmly persuaded that the fever was imported by the 'Eclair' and afterwards spread throughout the island by contagion from one person to another. I have taken considerable pains to trace out and discover the supposed morbid concatenation, but in vain. It becomes, therefore, a duty to express my opinion decidedly, that there is no satisfactory proof of the disease having been propagated by contagion, or from a specific poison which is said to emanate from the bodies of the sick, the dying, or the dead."

The case of the "Eclair," as has been already stated, is the one on which the greatest reliance is placed in proof of the importation of epidemic disease.

***

It is needful to advert to one instance more of alleged importation; namely, the introduction of the Yellow Fever epidemic of 1828 into the Garrison of Gibraltar by the ship "Dygden." This case has been more rigorously examined than any other, and on that account it exhibits a better specimen than can usually be obtained of the manner in which the evidence for these cases is commonly got up.

The most positive assertions having been made that this epidemic was introduced into Gibraltar by a ship from the Havannah, the "Dygden," the then Secretary of State for the Colonies, Sir George Murray, appointed a Special Commission to inquire into the facts of the case; consisting of the Judge Advocate, the Colonial or Civil Secretary, the Captain of the Port, and head of the quarantine department, the Town Major, or head of the police, the Principal Medical Officer of the garrison, and a Staff Surgeon. It was the desire of Sir George Murray that the Governor should act as president, on the ground that "as the proposed investigation is merely to ascertain a fact, it may be more properly accomplished by the careful examination of impartial witnesses than by the application of scientific research;" but Sir George Don, "not finding himself equal to the task," appointed, by desire of the Secretary of State, conveyed in a subsequent despatch, the British Superintendent of Quarantine, Sir William Pym, to preside in his place.

The facts alleged and attempted to be established before the Board with a view to prove that this epidemic was imported by the ship "Dygden" were, that this ship had arrived from the Havannah with Yellow Fever on board; that while in quarantine in the bay, she was visited from the garrison by a family of the name of Fenic, and that the first cases of the epidemic occurred in this family.

The first witness called to prove this alleged visit to the ship was a woman of the name of Villalunga, who stated that she lived in the yard of Fenic's house; that Fenic was a cigar-maker, that she assisted him in making cigars, that she heard the boy (Fenic's son) say that he, his sister, and his father had been on board the ship in the bay on Sunday, the day before the boy was taken ill, and that the boy told her that they had been on board "to eat, drink, and make merry," and "that his father had sold tobacco on board the ship."

The next witness brought forward was a child Caffiero, 11 years old, who stated that he was in the habit of playing with the two Fenics: that he lived very near them; that he played with them *every day before their death*, and that he saw them *every* day when they were sick in bed.

On these statements the Judge Advocate, Mr Howell, observes:—

"The only evidence which up to this period (April 10th) had been given to connect the illness in Fenic's family with a visit on ship-board, is the hearsay tale told by Villalunga, nor did she give to Fenic and his two children any companion in their alleged Sunday excursion." * *

"Eight days after his examination above mentioned, the boy Caffiero re-appears as a witness (viz., April 18th) with a story entirely new, and which, if credible, would be extremely material; because he affects to speak of facts which had before rested on the hearsay evidence of Villalunga, but of which facts Caffiero now, after the lapse of eight days, represents himself to have been an eye-witness. On this his re-appearance, however, he carefully abstains from giving any date, either day of the week, or month, or even season of the year. This cautious avoiding of dates may not unfairly be attributed to the variance between himself and Villalunga, in their respective journals of the illness of Fenic's children. Caffiero now says, 'I knew Salvo and Catalina Fenic, and went on board ship with them; *I do not recollect* the day. We went on board a three-masted ship. *I do not recollect* to what nation it belonged. We remained on deck and did not go below. We remained on board about one hour. Fenic, the father, took us on board; he rowed the boat himself; he ate and drank on board, and then brought *a bundle of clothes on shore.*'

"Until this time, neither he nor Villalunga said anything about a bundle of clothes.

"This boy's second evidence thus proceeds:—'I did not understand the language of the people on board the ship; they appeared to speak like Jews or Moors. I did not go on board more than once. When we landed on the wharf, the Maltese,' *i.e.* Fenic, '*gave me some money, a pistoreen, and told me not to say anything to anybody about our having been on board.*'

"The effect which this was designed to produce is obvious, viz., that the ship visited was in quarantine, and Fenic, the Maltese, was conscious that he had committed an offence against the quarantine laws which rendered it necessary for his own safety that he should bribe this boy to secrecy. This story is full of incongruities; it is not probable that a man should select for his Sunday excursion, to eat, drink, and make merry, a ship in quarantine; it is more improbable still that Fenic should gratuitously place himself in extreme peril, by taking with him (to be witnesses of his offence) children of the artless ages of 10, 11, and 13, on an expedition which, in his own judgment, as demonstrated by his own act, he is convinced exposes him to severe punishment.

"But with regard to the ship 'Dygden,' I find that she had already received pratique, and had been admitted to free intercourse with the shore, on the 6th of August, *four days previously to the alleged visit of Fenic,* the date of which, notwithstanding Caffiero's loss of memory on his second examination, had already been ascertained by Villalunga to have been Sunday, August 10th, on which day Fenic, therefore, could commit no crime by going on board; and the story of the bribe and injunction to secrecy resolves itself into a clumsy and ill-disguised attempt at giving a colour of guilt to a fabulous occurrence which, even if it had been real, would have been guiltless.

"His second evidence concludes thus:—'My mother was a washerwoman, and washed for a black woman who lived next her. Fenic's wife refused to wash the bundle of clothes that he brought ashore; he offered them to my mother, who also refused them; he then gave them to an Englishwoman: I knew her: *she is dead: I do not know her name, nor where she lived.*' I find by my notes that he added, 'This occurred during last winter,' although the words are not entered upon the minutes. He was then asked, 'What season of the year was it that you were on board of ship?' To which he cautiously replied, 'It was either summer or winter, I believe.'

"Evidence such as this, and given as I saw it given, bears on its face every character of falsehood; and disbelieving as I do this boy's whole story, and at the same time considering his extreme youth, the testimony given by him has upon my mind the further operation of tainting with more than suspicion all the other evidence proceeding from the same class of witnesses, which consisted chiefly of hearsay in conversation with persons who had since died; because it would seem that this child must have been an instrument in the hands of some one of maturer age."

The suspicion attached to the second appearance of this child is confirmed by a similar re-appearance of Villalunga, who, after sixteen days' absence from the Board, on the 24th of April, again presents herself as a witness. She now remembers that Mrs Fenic had asked her to wash some clothes; that she did not wash them, being herself indisposed; but that she was told by Mrs Fenic that she put these clothes out to be washed.

Mr Howell thus comments on this second appearance of Villalunga:—

"I have observed that Caffiero added to his original testimony so much as to give to it a new character altogether; I now observe that six days after Caffiero's amended testimony, and sixteen days after her own original examination, the woman Villalunga comes back with a new story, of which, singularly enough, the principal point is made to coincide with the alterations and emendations in the evidence of Caffiero."

On an examination of the surviving member of the Fenic family, the widow of Fenic himself, it appears that she gave a positive denial to this alleged visit of her husband and children to the ship.

"She was at my desire," says Mr Howell, "particularly reminded that the duty which she owed to society required her to disclose everything that she knew; and from the ingenuous manner in which her evidence was given, I am led to believe that she spoke the truth.

"She declared that she did not know the cause of her children's illness:—
'They were attended by Dr Lopez, who is dead, and who said they had a
tabardillo and indigestion, *caused by eating green figs*. He did not say what was
the cause of the tabardillo. My husband was a cigar-maker; but he did not
go on board ship either to buy tobacco or to sell cigars. Neither my
husband nor my children went into the bay at any time during last summer
or autumn. I know this: because if they had gone, they would have told me,
and they did not tell me.' Nor, indeed, is it to be supposed that the children
would not have told their mother, and that the husband would not have
told his wife, that which all of them are declared to have communicated so
freely to other people."

On being cited before a Public Notary at Gibraltar (November 14th,
1829), this witness still more particularly deposed—

"That it was utterly untrue that her husband went on board any ship in
the bay at any time last summer; that on account of his age and infirmity, he
had not been in a boat for ten years past; that she is equally certain that her
two children never went on board any boat or ship; that, with respect to the
boy Caffiero, neither she nor any of her family knew anything about him;
and that his story of having gone on board the ship with her husband and
her two children, 'is a made-up falsehood.'"

Mr Howell sums up the result of his examination of the evidence
adduced before the Board respecting the Fenic family in the following
words:—

"Having thus examined in detail the evidence adduced to connect the
illness of Salvador Fenic (the alleged first case of the epidemic) with the
'Dygden,'—and no other vessel has been pointed at,—I find not only that
it completely fails to make out even a *primâ facie* case, but also, from the
whole complexion of the evidence, I am convinced that the story of Fenic's
visit to that vessel on the 10th of August is, from beginning to end, a
fabrication."

Apparently in anticipation of a failure to connect the illness in Fenic's
family with a foreign source, much testimony was given before the Board
derived, as is stated by Mr Howell, "through channels most impure," about
instances in which foul clothes are supposed to have been brought ashore
by sailors arriving from the Havannah, in the early part of the epidemic,
and which foul clothes infected the washerwomen.

After showing at some length the discrepancies and contradictions
which proved the whole testimony adduced on this point to be utterly
worthless, Mr Howell says:—

"Here I leave the journals of washerwomen, and the tattle of their gossips, remarking this fatal objection to each washing-tub anecdote, however circumstantial, that *not one of them goes back so far as to precede*, and therefore to account for, *the alleged first case of the epidemic*, namely, that of Salvador Fenic, who, as we are told, fell ill *on the 11th of August*, and upon whose single case, therefore, the proof of importation rests. And if the attempt to connect the illness of Salvador Fenic with a foreign source be, as I hold it to be, a complete failure, how is the illness of the boy Caffiero to be accounted for? And to what is to be ascribed the illness of Mr Martin's child on August 16th, a case quite as early as that of Caffiero, and which has not been attempted to be traced to importation? not one of the washing-tub cases being anterior either to that of Mr Martin's child or to that of Caffiero, both of which are unquestioned cases of the epidemic."

It was essential to the proof of the connection of the "Dygden" with the outbreak of the epidemic, to establish the fact of the existence of Yellow Fever on board the ship. No proof of this appears to have been adduced. On the contrary, the captain of the ship declares that no such disease existed on board; the head of the Quarantine Department, after an official examination into the fact, affirms that there is no evidence whatever to disprove the truth of the captain's statement, and the Quarantine Medical Officer, after "a minute inspection of the captain and crew," states that he "found them all in perfect health."

"I have minutely inspected the captain and crew," he says, "whom I found in perfect health. The reason for putting this ship in quarantine for 40 days was, that two men died on the passage. It is now 66 clear days since the first man died, and 61 since the death of the last, and nothing like disease has since appeared, nor have I the most distant reason to apprehend danger to the public health from any circumstances connected with the 'Dygden.'"

Mr Howell calls special attention to this report of the medical officer:—

"This report," he says, "was written, as it strikes me, under circumstances which entitle it to much consideration. This ship had been officially pointed out to him (as the Medical Officer of Quarantine) as being strongly suspected. The responsibility of his office was thus brought fully before his eyes, and he had *then* no motive for making a false report of his inspection of the 'Dygden's' master and crew, because the epidemic had not at that period commenced. If he had observed any reasonable grounds for suspicion, he had only to fall in with the rumour, and recommend that none of the persons or susceptible articles on board should be permitted to land. The conduct and declarations, therefore, of Dr Hennen, as a responsible public officer, under such circumstances, when, if he erred at all, it would probably be on the side of *over caution*, I hold to be most material."

Such is a fair specimen of the evidence adduced on this occasion to establish a positive case of importation. It breaks down at every point. There is complete failure in the proof that Yellow Fever existed on board the ship; there is complete failure in the proof that there was the slightest connection between the ship and any persons on shore; and there is even failure in the proof that the individuals who are alleged to have introduced the disease were really affected with a malady of the same nature as the epidemic that subsequently prevailed.

The Judge Advocate thus states the conclusion at which he arrived after a careful examination of the proceedings of the Commission:—

"I am of opinion that the evidence brought forward has totally failed to prove that the late epidemic disease was introduced from any foreign source, either by the Swedish ship 'Dygden' or by any other means; and I am further of opinion that the late epidemic had its origin in Gibraltar."

Medical observers on the spot, not members of the Board, but who carefully watched its proceedings, it is believed, without any exception, arrived at the same conclusion. Thus Dr T. Smith sums up the result of his examination of the subject in the following words:—

"That it was not imported I think every candid man will admit who has deliberately weighed the evidence given on the subject before the Board of Commissioners, and the facts I have stated. Every endeavour to establish the importation doctrine has failed, and both the Colonial Secretary, Sir George Murray, and Sir James McGrigor, Director-General of the Army Medical Department, I have heard, are convinced there is not the slightest ground for such a belief; but, on the contrary, that there is every reason to suppose the disease owed its origin to causes within the walls of the garrison."

Several comments were made by those who paid attention to the subject at the time, on the manner in which this investigation was conducted, which appear to deserve notice.

Complaints were made that the result of the inquiry was prejudged. In proof of this it was found that the President of the Board, a few days before it held its first meeting, addressed to the military secretary of the garrison an official letter in which, among other observations directly tending to a prejudgment of the case, he affirms, that "the fever in question has often been traced to importation, and against this source *only* must we look for its prevention."

It appears further that before the meeting of the Board an official intimation of the views and wishes of the local authorities was promulgated in the Government Gazette, into which nothing is admitted but by authority, in the following words:—

"The scourge from which we have been by Divine Providence just delivered must be an exotic of some kind. It is in its origin independent of everything inherent in the soil which we inhabit, incapable of existing among us during the winter months, and totally distinct from and unconnected with the Remitting and Intermitting Fever, which may be said to be unknown in this garrison."

"Two causes," observes Mr Howell, "concurred to operate injuriously upon the proceedings of the Board: *First*, the conviction universally prevalent among the *civil* population of Gibraltar, that the prosperity of that community would be undermined if it should be proved that the epidemic had been generated on the spot, because of the prohibitions and restrictions which it was anticipated would in that case be inflicted upon its commercial intercourse with other places. Hence the notion that not only the last epidemic, but that all its predecessors had been imported from some foreign country was not only anxiously supported by the unanimous voice of the civil community, but it was with equal unanimity believed that a different doctrine would be fatal to the commercial prosperity of the place. From this feeling of self-interest it is to be admitted that the *military* were exempt, a distinction between the two classes which ought to be taken into account in estimating the value of the evidence taken by the Board, and more especially the evidence of the medical practitioners.

"The *second* cause operating injuriously upon this inquiry was the publication, in the official government newspaper (into which nothing is admitted except by official authority), on January 12, 1829, of an article authoritatively announcing that the late epidemic had been imported into Gibraltar, and denouncing as void of common sense any person who should hold a different opinion. This official notification of the feelings of the local Government (preceding as it did by only 12 days the appointment of the Board of Inquiry) could hardly fail to encourage evidence on one side, and discourage evidence on the other."

Complaints were also made that there was a partial selection of witnesses.

"It always appeared most extraordinary and 'unjustifiable,'" says Dr Gillkrest, "that on this kind of inquiry, which was intended by the Secretary of State to be so beneficial to the interests of humanity, the Superintendent of Quarantine, as president, should have assumed the right in several instances of selecting the witnesses, which obviously prejudiced the question, and by which much of the truth was intercepted.

"Several medical officers of the garrison who had much experience respecting the progress of the epidemic, were either not examined at all, or only in a very imperfect manner. I was among the latter, being surgeon to the 43rd Regiment, and present during the whole epidemic. After a very limited examination, I officially informed the President, by letter, that I had much to state; but, like others, I was not called afterwards.

"From what I felt due to the service of which I had been a member for so many years, as well as the cause of truth, I was induced to protest against such proceedings, which protest will, I presume, be found with the documents connected with the inquiry forwarded from Gibraltar to the Colonial Office in London."

Complaints were further made of the mode of collecting the evidence adopted on this occasion, which was such as to excite the suspicion of some of the members of the Commission, and to lead eventually to their condemnation of it, and their repudiation of the Report which was founded upon it.[38]

38. *See* Letter of Sir George Murray, and reply of Colonel Chapman, the Civil Secretary, p. 274;—also Report of Judge Howell, Second Report on Quarantine of the General Board of Health, Appendix II., pp. 245, 273.

APPENDIX

A return of the Sanitary Works carried out in those towns to which the Public Health Act has been applied, was laid on the table of the House of Commons, on the 12th of April last, and ordered to be printed (No. 176, Session 1866). In view of the threatened Epidemic, however, the unusual labour cast upon the Local Government Office,—now charged with the superintendence of Local Boards of Health,—must render it improbable that time can be found to examine the proof of this important return before the end of the Session.

At this still early period in the progress of Sanitary Reform, any such return must be manifestly imperfect; yet it will probably be found that ten times the sum mentioned in the text[39] is already known to have been expended on these works; and previous returns show that about a million and a half sterling has, in addition, been laid out in the provision of Extramural Cemeteries.

39. See p. 57.

The effect of these measures, in reducing the mortality of the population, cannot of course be calculated at present with any degree of accuracy; because no statistics of this nature can be reliable, unless based upon an average of many years. It will, nevertheless, be exceedingly interesting to watch the results of these improvements in the civilization of England; improvements which have been, perhaps, mainly effected by the labours of Dr Southwood Smith.

That such Sanitary appliances are not yet all that could be wished in many of our larger towns, is abundantly exhibited by the following extract from the Quarterly Report of the Registrar-General for January, February, and March, 1866.

"If the map of England were shaded to represent the rates of mortality of last quarter in the registration districts, the eye, travelling from the lighter south to the darker north, would be instantly drawn to a spot of portentous darkness on the Mersey; and the question would be asked whether cholera, the black death, or other plague, imported with bales of merchandise, had been lately introduced into its busy and populous seaport. Happily this has not been the case; but fever, probably developed or aided by the mild and damp atmosphere of the season, and by overcrowding in an increasing population, has been busy and fatal in Liverpool, and in other towns of the same county and of Yorkshire. The annual mortality of the borough of

Liverpool in the three months was excessive, and demands immediate and earnest consideration; it rose to 4.593 per cent. This implies that if this death-rate were maintained for a year, 46 persons out of 1000 in the population would die in that time, or 15 more than died in Glasgow, its northern rival, 19 more than in London. The mortality in the city of Manchester, though far less than that of Liverpool, was higher than in any other of the 13 selected towns of the United Kingdom; it was 3.742 per cent.; and that of Leeds was hardly less."

THE END